POLICY AND PRACTICE IN
NUMBER FIFTEEN

Alcohol

POLICY AND PRACTICE IN HEALTH AND SOCIAL CARE

POLICY AND PRACTICE IN HEALTH AND SOCIAL CARE

SERIES EDITORS

JOYCE CAVAYE and ALISON PETCH

Alcohol

Ken Barrie

Senior Lecturer in Alcohol and Drug Studies
University of the West of Scotland

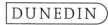

For Nancy

Published by
Dunedin Academic Press Ltd
Hudson House
8 Albany Street
Edinburgh EH1 3QB
Scotland

ISBN: 978–1–906716–31–8
ISSN: 1750–1407

First published 2012
© 2012 Ken Barrie

British Library Cataloguing in Publication data
A catalogue record for this book is available from the British Library

Typeset by Makar Publishing Production
Printed in Great Britain by CPI Antony Rowe

CONTENTS

SERIES EDITORS' INTRODUCTION

Discussion of alcohol is omnipresent, a topic of conversation beloved of the media, politicians and people in the street alike. Opinions and advice abound and the individual seeking to make sense of it all can be lost in a morass of apparently conflicting ideas and recommendations. This volume seeks to distinguish fact from fiction and evidence from speculation to provide a sober assessment of the role of alcohol in our lives, and most particularly within the culture of Scottish life.

An opening chapter sets the scene, exploring what is meant by safe drinking and when consumption will be defined as hazardous, harmful or at binge level. Current levels of consumption are discussed, distinguished by demographic factors, and challenging some of the assumptions in widespread circulation. The health, social and economic consequences of excessive consumption are then identified, highlighting for example alcohol dependence in 6% of the Scottish population and healthcare costs estimated to be in the order of £269 million.

The third chapter addresses the contentious issue of alcohol pricing, exploring the extent to which variation in price impacts on consumption of different drinks and hence on health-related consequences. This is followed by a similar analysis of the variations by place of consumption and the associated potential for regulation of the drinking environment.

The focus of the final chapters switches to the most effective strategies and treatments for those already experiencing the negative consequences of their drinking. The concept of recovery is explored, identifying the triggers for change and the options for staying free from harm. The evidence for the effectiveness of different approaches is elegantly distilled and case studies illustrate potentially different routes to recovery. Finally, a range of different options in the form of Alcohol Brief Interventions (ABIs) and specialist treatment are addressed through a rigorous exploration of the evidence base.

We learnt a lot from editing this volume; we hope our readers will also.

Dr Joyce Cavaye
Faculty of Health and Social Care, The Open University in Scotland, Edinburgh

Professor Alison Petch
The Institute for Research and Innovation in Social Services (IRISS), Glasgow

ACKNOWLEDGEMENTS

For their encouragement, Alison Fitzpatrick, Dougie Marks, Iain McPhee, Linda Cusick at Alcohol and Drug Studies, University of the West of Scotland.

GLOSSARY OF ABBREVIATIONS

AA	Alcoholics Anonymous
ABI	alcohol brief interventions
ABV	alcohol by volume
AFS	Alcohol Focus Scotland
ARBD	alcohol-related brain damage
ANARP	Alcohol needs assessment research project
ATTC	Addiction Technology Transfer Center
AUDIT	alcohol use disorders identification test
BASW	British Association of Social Workers
BI	brief interventions
BMI	brief motivational interviewing
BMJ	British Medical Journal
CAGE	Have you ever felt you should **C**ut down on your drinking? Have people **A**nnoyed you by criticising your drinking? Have you ever felt bad or **G**uilty? Have you ever had a drink first thing in the morning (**E**ye opener)?
CBI	combine behavioural intervention
CBT	cognitive behavioural therapy
COSLA	Convention of Scottish Local Authorities
CPRS	Central Policy Review Staff
DHSS	Department of Health and Social Security
DOH	Department of Health
DVLA	Driver Vehicle Licensing Authority
FAS	foetal alcohol syndrome
FAST	fast alcohol screening test
FRAMES	**F**eedback: on risk and harm from screening, assessment or test; **R**esponsibility: emphasis on personal responsibility for alcohol use and change; **A**dvice: provision of clear practical advice and

	self-help material; **M**enu: options for change; **E**mpathy: non-judgemental and supportive; **S**elf-efficacy: increase individual's belief in their ability to change
FPN	fixed penalty notice
GCPH	Glasgow Centre for Population Health
GGT	gamma glutamyl transferase
GHS	General Household Survey
HTBS	Health Technology Board for Scotland
ICD	International Classification of Diseases
IHD	ischaemic heart disease
ISD	Information Services Division
MATCH	matching alcoholism treatment and client heterogeneity
MCV	mean corpuscular volume
MET	motivational enhancement therapy
NA	Narcotics Anonymous
NCD	non-communicable disease
NIAAA	National Institute on Alcohol Abuse and Alcoholism
NICE	National Institute for Clinical Excellence
NNT	numbers needed to treat
NTA	National Treatment Agency (England and Wales)
NTORS	National Treatment Outcome Research Study
ONS	Office for National Statistics
OPCS	Office of Population Censuses and Surveys
PAT	Paddington alcohol test
PRIME	prospective study of myocardial infarction
RCT	randomised controlled trial
RPI	retail price index
SALSUS	schools adolescent lifestyle and substance-use survey
SBNT	social behaviour network therapy
SIGN	Scottish inter-collegiate guidelines network
SMACAP	Scottish ministerial advisory committee on alcohol problems
SMR	standardised all-cause mortality ratios
T-ACE	**T**ake number of drinks, **A**nnoyed, **C**ut down, **E**ye Opener

TSF	Twelve Step Facilitation
TTM	trans-theoretical model
TWEAK	Tolerance, Worried, Eye Opener, Amnesia, Kut down
UKATT	United Kingdom alcohol treatment trial, 2008
WHO	World Health Organization

INTRODUCTION

Alcohol is Scotland's favourite psychoactive drug, just as it is in every other European country and many others besides. Production, sale and export of alcohol are major elements of the economy. Consumption and problems are currently at their highest in the UK for quite some time and significantly higher still in Scotland. However, a modest reduction in consumption and consequences, in recent years, may be associated with the economic downturn.

The overall aim of this book is to consider alcohol-related problems, in Scotland, in the early twenty-first century, and to adopt a 'what works' approach to how these problems may be reduced based on the international research evidence. As a result, some commonly debated themes have been omitted: 'alcohol education' because there is little evidence that such approaches reduce alcohol-related harm in their own right; and alcohol advertising because the rapid technological developments in communication make many evidence-informed proposals to control advertising redundant, though advertising successfully influences attitudes among young people, which are predictive of drinking later in life.

Scottish governments, since devolution in 1999, have paid considerable attention to the problems associated with alcohol and made significant inroads into implementing their proposals, perhaps more vigorously than in other parts of the UK. The Licensing (Scotland) Act 2005 has a clear objective — to consider public health — making it unique in the UK. The Scottish Government published the Alcohol (Minimum Pricing) Bill in November 2011 and MSPs were urged to offer their support. Substantial developments have taken place in embedding 'brief interventions' into healthcare practice. Proposed changes to the devolution agreement, if approved, would allow the Scottish Parliament to reduce the drink driving legal limit.

Scottish drinking habits and associated harms will be considered in the context of the UK. From a policy perspective the potential to alter alcohol-related harm by price regulation and to control the drinking environment via liquor licensing will be evaluated. At an individual level the potential to resolve alcohol problems will be examined and placed in the context of health and social policy. The evidence for recovery, with or without access to specialist treatment, and brief interventions will be elaborated upon.

This book should be of relevance to all who have an interest in health and social sciences, whether as researchers, policymakers or healthcare providers and practitioners. It may also interest those with an interest in the diversity of responses to alcohol problems available within a devolved government framework. However, there's little point in being parochial, quite the reverse, and there's a wealth of research evidence to consider.

CHAPTER 1

Drinking in the UK

Freedom and whisky gang thegither. (Robert Burns)

The European region is the heaviest drinking region in the world, with over one fifth of the population of 15 years old and over, reporting heavy episodic drinking at least once a week. Heavy episodic drinking is widespread across all ages and all of Europe. (WHO, 2010)

Drinking is influenced by a wide range of economic, social and psychological factors. This chapter will outline how alcohol consumption is measured and how consumption levels are associated with levels of alcohol-related problems. Consideration will be given to the factors that influence per capita consumption of alcohol in the UK. Consumption levels and drinking patterns, drawn from surveys, will be examined through the influences of age, gender and social background, as well as regional and national differences. There will be a focus on Scottish drinking habits.

Alcohol is the UK's most commonly used psychoactive drug. The use of alcohol is embedded in UK culture for the purposes of celebration, ranging from marking the end of the working week to weddings and other formal occasions. It is also used to commiserate. As alcohol has become cheaper and more accessible more opportunities to drink have become available. Broadly speaking, the drinking population in the UK is interested in the intoxicating effects of alcohol, including the occasional and sometimes regular pursuit of drunkenness, achieved by so-called binge drinking. Despite the majority of those over the age of sixteen being 'drinkers' there is considerable variation in alcohol consumption associated with social background, ethnicity and national and regional differences.

Measuring drinking and guidance on consumption

From brewing and distillation processes a wide range of alcoholic beverages are produced ranging in strength from low alcohol beers at 1% alcohol by volume (ABV) to 'cask strength' spirits at around 60% ABV, with many in between. Irrespective of the production method or type of beverage a 'unit' of alcohol is 10g of pure alcohol (ethanol). Table 1.1 outlines the unit equivalent in relation to ABV of alcoholic beverages commonly sold in the UK, the number of units commonly found in a bottle and variations commonly found in ABV, depending on strength in the same beverage.

Table 1.1: Units of alcohol and ABV in common beverages and bottle sizes.

Beverage	Unit equivalent	ABV	Bottle: units	Variations in ABV
Beer	0.5pt (235 ml) of 'ordinary strength' beer	3.5–4%	50cl: 2–3	5–7% ABV is common
Cider	0.5pt (235 ml) of 'ordinary strength' cider	3.5–4%	200cl: 8–16	6–8% ABV is common
Table wine	Small glass of table wine (125ml)	9–10%	70cl: 6–9	12–13% ABV is common
Fortified wine	35ml measure	15–20%	70cl: 11–14	Some contain caffeine
Spirits	25ml measure	40%	70cl: 28	Often sold in 35ml measures

Measuring alcohol consumption on the basis of units is complicated by the extent to which many beverages (beer, cider, wine) are available in higher ABV than the 'unit equivalent'. Table wines are commonly 12–13% ABV and beers and ciders are commonly available at 6% and 8% ABV respectively, so it is possible that for some beverages the same volume of a particular alcoholic beverage , e.g. table wine may contain up to 50% more ABV. Some fortified wines — often labelled as 'tonic' wines — contain caffeine, and while this may change the effect of the beverage it does not alter the ABV. Spirits are sold in licensed premises in 25ml measures (one unit); however, in

Scotland 35ml measures are common, 40% greater alcohol content than the standard 'unit' used in UK drinking surveys. Some of these variations have been incorporated into updating the measurement of alcohol consumption, in population surveys since 2008 (Robinson et al., 2011). This attempted to capture the move towards the sale of wine in larger glasses as well as the wide range of higher-strength beverages now available. No adjustment has been made for the variation in spirit measures in Scotland.

Table 1.2: Recommended drinking guidelines.

Drinking	Men	Women
Daily		
Recommended/'safe' daily*	3–4 units maximum	2–3 units maximum
Pregnancy		0 units daily; 1–2 units maximum
Binge: daily amounts	More than 8 units	More than 6 units
Weekly		
Recommended/'safe' weekly	21 units maximum	14 units maximum
Hazardous	22+ units	15+ units
Harmful	50+ units	36+ units

* Recommended or 'safer' consumption suggests that drinkers should refrain from drinking on two days per week.

UK government and health authorities have set out recommended alcohol consumption levels for men and women in an attempt to inform the public, influence alcohol consumption and reduce levels of consumption, which have the potential to result in harm (hazardous drinking) or which do in fact cause harm (harmful drinking) (DOH, 1995). Given the detail outlined in Table 1.2 it is not surprising to find that accurate recollection of the guidance on alcohol consumption is limited.

Recommended limits

Health guidance in the UK recommends that men and women should drink no more than twenty-one and fourteen units of alcohol per week, respectively. On a daily basis this amounts to 3–4 units per day for men and 2–3 units per day for women, with two alcohol-free days per week. There are different views on drinking during pregnancy ranging from advice to abstain from alcohol to the suggestion of a maximum of 1–2 units of alcohol per day, once or twice a week (Burns *et al.*, 2010). However, all UK chief medical officers advise that women who are pregnant or trying to conceive should avoid alcohol (Scottish Government, 2008c).

Consumption levels
Abstinence
In 2009 85% of adults were alcohol consumers, ranging from light/occasional to harmful: 12% men and 18% women were abstainers. Around 30% of men and 40% of women in both England and Scotland had not had an alcoholic drink in the previous week (Bromley and Shelton, 2010).

Levels of abstinence were at their greatest among women aged more than sixty-five years. Only 10% of men in the 25–64 age group were abstainers. Some reported that they had always been a non-drinker (57%) and 43% reported that they had given up drinking. Among those who had never drank, almost half said they did not like it, whilst more than a quarter stated religious reasons. Of those who had given up drinking, more than half stated health reasons and just over one-fifth indicated that they did not like it (Robinson et al., 2011).

Hazardous drinking
Men drinking in excess of twenty-one units and women drinking in excess of fourteen units of alcohol per week are considered to be drinking hazardously. Those males who drink in excess of eight units per day and women drinking in excess of six units per day are also considered to be 'at risk' even if they do not exceed the weekly safe drinking limit. These limits offer one definition of binge drinking. Hazardous drinking relates to the risk or potential for harm or negative consequences to result, irrespective of whether they actually occur. A male who drinks four pints (eight units) of beer per day, for example, may not directly experience any problems; however, risks are attached either in the short or longer term e.g. accidents and chronic health problems.

Hazardous drinking is not a diagnostic term and is defined by WHO (1994) as a pattern of substance use that increases the risk of harmful consequences to the user. In contrast to harmful use hazardous use refers to patterns of use that are of public health significance despite the absence of any current disorder in the individual. The proportion of those men and women consuming in excess of four/ three units per day reflected government advice on recommended limits for alcohol consumption. Among men 37% and among women 20% exceeded the recommended intake. Hazardous drinkers are commonly identified through screening programmes in general healthcare. They are likely to be offered alcohol brief interventions (ABI) (see Chapter 6).

Harmful drinking

Men consuming in excess of fifty units per week, or eight units per day, and women in excess of thirty-five units per week, or six units per day are considered harmful drinkers. They will often have clear signs of alcohol-related damage (WHO, 1993) and a significant proportion are likely to be moderately to severely dependent on alcohol (Raistrick et al., 2006). Among men 20% drank harmfully and 13% of women drank harmfully. When broken down by age heavy or harmful drinking was noted more commonly in both younger men and women (Robinson et al., 2011). However, in Scotland a significantly lower proportion of men drank within the recommended guidelines (up to four units per day) when compared to men in England. Furthermore, Scottish men were more likely to drink in excess of these limits. Average consumption on heavy drinking days was almost 50% higher (6.2 and 4.3 units) among Scottish men, when compared with English men.

A significantly lower proportion of women drank within the recommended guidelines (up to three units per day) in Scotland compared to England. Average consumption on heavy drinking days was in excess of 50% higher (3.5 and 2.2 units) among Scottish women, when compared with English women. Consumption among women in Scotland, unlike men, was on average in excess of the recommended limits (2–3 units). In Scotland and England 18% and 15% of women, respectively, drank harmfully (more than six units on heaviest drinking day). In both England and Scotland significant proportions of men and women had drunk hazardously and harmfully in the previous seven days. Levels of both hazardous and harmful alcohol consumption were noted to be higher in Scotland (Bromley and Shelton, 2010).

Binge drinking

> 'We never called it binge drinking. It was the weekend.'
> (focus group respondent, McPhee, 2011)

There is no commonly agreed definition of binge drinking (Marks *et al.*, 2011) and this is reflected in public perception of the term. The term 'binge drinking' is a recent term which reflects a style of drinking common not only to Scottish drinking culture but also to the rest of the UK. The plan for action on alcohol (Scottish Executive, 2002) defines binge drinking as 'drinking an excessive amount on any one occasion'. However, it is known that men and women are likely to suffer alcohol-related consequences when regularly drinking in excess of eight units and six units respectively on a heavy drinking day (Robinson et al., 2011) and this measure has become the convention in UK population surveys. The essence of binge drinking is a pattern of high consumption, in a relatively short period of time, thereby maximising the intoxicating effects of alcohol. However, by merely paying attention to the amount consumed, on a daily basis, the nature of binge drinking goes unnoticed. If an individual consumes ten units of alcohol starting at midday, for example, and consumes one unit per hour, she or he would be very unlikely to have a blood alcohol measure over 20mg alcohol per 100ml blood (where, for example, the legal limit for drink driving is 80mg alcohol per 100ml blood). Whilst a large amount of alcohol may be consumed on one drinking day the pattern of consumption can hardly be described as a 'binge' given that a high blood alcohol level is never achieved and 'drunken behaviour' is not apparent. It may be that a more subjective measure, such as reporting 'feeling drunk' or 'feeling very drunk' is a better indicator of binge drinking (SALSUS, 2008).

Many harmful drinkers are binge drinkers, as their drinking pattern consists of regular high-volume drinking days, most of which could be described as a 'binge', as distinct from 'risky single-occasion' drinkers, where high consumption is irregular, or perhaps weekly

(Gmel *et al.*, 2011). The persistent high-volume, serial binge drinking of the harmful drinker tends to result in chronic health and social consequences, whereas the risky single-occasion drinker will more commonly experience problems associated with accidents and social disorder.

In a study of further and higher education students in Scotland, Marks *et al.* (2011) interviewed more than 300 students (mean age twenty-three, range 16–58 years), of whom 80% were female and 65% of the sample fitted criteria for binge drinking. This style of alcohol consumption, given the large proportion of the sample fitting the criteria, is normal in Scottish culture. When binge drinkers were compared with non-binge drinkers no differences in ethnicity, social class, employment status or gender were found. However, binge drinkers were more likely to report drinking to be sociable, to conform, to forget worries and for excitement. They also reported higher levels of alcohol-related consequences, stress and depression and having started drinking at an earlier age. Frequency of hangovers predicted symptoms of depression (Paljarva *et al.*, 2009).

Expenditure and sales

The expenditure in the UK for 2000 on alcohol was £38.5 billion, rising to a peak of £44.4 billion in 2004 and falling subsequently to £37 billion in 2009, at constant 2006 prices. In Scotland for the same year, total sales were worth £3.64 billion reflecting a 9% increase from 2005. During the period 2005–9 on-trade sales increased by 1% while sales at off-trade establishments increased by 22%. Modest decreases in beer and spirit sales were outstripped by increases in sales of wine and cider. Between 2005 and 2009 there were reductions of less than 1% of total consumer expenditure on all alcoholic beverages in the UK. Per capita consumption of alcohol is measured in litres of pure alcohol, irrespective of the type of beverage and in the UK in 1947 was 3.5 litres per head of the population (House of Commons Health Committee, 2010).

In Scotland between 2005 and 2009 litres of pure alcohol sold remained fairly constant at twelve litres per annum per head of the population over the age of sixteen. During the same period around ten litres of pure alcohol were sold per head of the population in

England and Wales. This indicates that alcohol sales in Scotland are 20% greater per head of the population than in the rest of the UK. Across the UK the downturn in on-trade sales and the upturn in off-trade sales records are consistent with expenditure receipts for the same period. Similarly in Scotland in 2005 40% of sales were on-trade compared with 60% off-trade; by 2009 this had shifted to 30% and 70% respectively (ISD, 2011).

Population surveys

It is generally recognised that social surveys of drinking behaviour report lower levels of consumption than records from the sale of alcohol. This may be due to individuals consciously, or otherwise, underestimating their consumption, whether related to poor memory or a reluctance to divulge personal information. Memory of the detail of recent drinking may also lead to underestimation, particularly if a large amount has been consumed. It may also be due to the difficulty in estimating 'home poured' drinks, which tend to be larger than the measures served in licensed premises. As far as sampling is concerned it may also be that those heaviest alcohol consumers are not available, or do not wish to participate in such surveys.

Drinking surveys provide information that sales records cannot show, namely population accounts of alcohol consumption in relation to volume and frequency of drinking. In addition, they provide information on associations between individual characteristics, such as age, gender, socio-economic classification, region of residence and alcohol consumption, all of which may provide data required for the development of policy responses (Robinson et al., 2011; ISD, 2011). The best picture of alcohol consumption is based on a range of sources including both survey data and sales records.

Survey trends mid 1990s–2009: UK adults
1998–2000
During the 1990s the General Household Survey (GHS) reported a slight increase in consumption among men and a significantly greater increase among women. Following an increase between 1998 and 2000, a decline emerged in the hazardous drinking in men

(29% to 23%) and women (17% to 12%). Surveys show little change between 1998 and 2003, a period of peak consumption, based on reported previous seven days drinking or drinking in excess of recommended limits. A similar pattern emerged for harmful drinking by men and women, who exceeded eight/six units on at least one day per week.

2000–2006
Hazardous drinking in both men and women reduced between 2000 and 2006. This reduction was most noticeable in the 16–24 age group among men from 50% to 39%, and women from 42% to 34%. The proportion of men drinking harmfully also reduced from 37% to 27%.

2006/7–2009
More modest reductions were reported for 2007–9 and this downward shift in consumption continued and were reflected in alcohol sales data. There were reductions in the proportion of those reporting having had an alcoholic drink in the previous seven days: 72% to 68% of men; and 57% to 54% of women. Hazardous drinking among men reduced from 41% to 37% and from 34% to 29% among women. In respect of harmful drinking there were reductions from 23% to 20% (men) and 15% to 13% (women).

From consumption levels which were at their highest at the turn of the century, there has been a downward trend in consumption since around 2005/6, which is confirmed by surveys and sales data. This may in part be a result of the current economic downturn.

National and regional differences in alcohol consumption
Table 1.3 shows the average reported weekly consumption of men and women in Wales, Scotland and England, with further detail from English regions in 2009. Despite national stereotypes there were no significant differences between average weekly alcohol consumption between the countries of the UK. As far as England was concerned, the highest average weekly consumption was in the North-east (14.4 units) and the lowest in London (9.3 units) and a similar low in the West Midlands.

Table 1.3: Average weekly adult alcohol consumption (in units) by gender, country and English region.

Country	Average weekly consumption		
	Total	**Men**	**Women**
Wales	12.4	16.7	8.6
Scotland	11.2	15.0	7.8
England	11.9	16.4	8.0
English region			
North-east	14.4	21.0	9.4
North-west	13.1	17.3	9.0
Yorkshire and Humber	13.6	17.7	9.8
East Midlands	11.9	16.3	7.8
West Midlands	10.2	14.0	6.9
East of England	11.6	15.8	7.8
London	9.3	13.4	6.0
South-east	12.5	17.1	8.4
South-west	12.2	17.6	7.9
UK total	11.9	16.3	8.0

Source: Robinson *et al.*, 2011

In 2009, 69% of men and 55% of women in England consumed alcohol in the previous week compared to 58% and 48% respectively in Scotland. Men in Wales and England were more likely than men in Scotland to have an alcoholic drink on at least five days out of the previous seven days (17% and 19% compared with 12%). In the North-east, North-west and Yorkshire and Humber region the highest proportions of adults drinking in excess of four/three units (40%, 39% and 41%) were noted. They also showed the highest levels of heavy drinking resulting in their being the highest consuming regions in the UK.

On the basis of reported average weekly alcohol consumption Scotland does not stand out, consuming less than Wales and all English regions with the exceptions of London and the West Midlands. This appears to be contradicted by sales records of 20% higher per capita sales and consumption in Scotland compared to England (ISD, 2011). There seems to be considerable regional variations and these are more marked than national distinctions.

Children and young people's drinking

In a culture where alcohol is highly acceptable children are social-
ised into the drinking culture when they are quite young, long
before they actually consume alcohol. At a young age children have
a concept of alcohol and can distinguish between 'alcohol' bottles
and other drinks bottles at the age of four, and at the age of six, on
seeing film of a person staggering, will conclude that they are drunk,
as opposed to unwell. The family are the main source of influence
on younger children, followed by peer groups and media influences
as the young person moves into adolescence. Many parents give
young children sips of diluted alcoholic drinks as part of the belief
that home is the best place to learn about alcohol, based on their
own experiences of alcohol, rather than health messages. Despite
this, when asked parents are more likely to suggest that mid teens
is the best time to introduce young people to alcohol (Valentine
et al., 2010). However, parents may not be the best role models all
the time, and in some instances a heavy drinking parent may have
a negative impact on the child's understanding of drinking. Eadie
et al. (2010) indicate that there is a dynamic and complex series of
parent–child interactions regarding alcohol, rather than one way
from parent to child. As in many other matters, the family unit
ensures the transfer of culturally approved attitudes and behaviours
regarding alcohol. As parental influence decreases and as young
people move into early adolescence, Percy *et al.* (2011) describes an
'implicit contract' between parent and child, whereby parents know
about the young person's drinking but do not necessarily need to
see the young person intoxicated. One strategy adopted by young
people is to drink to the required level earlier in the evening and to
return home more sober. Further attempts to restrict drinking may
be resisted and in some instances parental actions may increase the
likelihood of drunkenness. However, evidence of family instability
and of excessive drinking itself in a parent, or parents, may result
in more extreme attitudes and behaviour in the younger person,
either in favour of excessive drinking or abstinence (Sondhi and
Turner, 2011).

Drinking confers social standing and peer acceptance, making
the struggle to cope with initially unpleasant tasting drinks

worthwhile. In line with peer acceptance, young people were more likely to admit to drinking recently, and to certain amounts of alcohol, if most of their friends did too. Young people tend to drink to get drunk, described as a culture of intoxication, despite most parental influences supporting moderation. Drinking and getting drunk are therefore skills, strongly reinforced by the peer culture, whereby achieving the desired level of intoxication is balanced with the need to sober up in time to go home. However, young people do not have a drinking culture which is entirely unique and disconnected from parents and the broader adult drinking culture.

Surveys of young peoples' drinking, under the age of sixteen, are usually conducted on school students. Among thirteen and fifteen year olds in Scotland, 52% and 82% respectively indicated that they had 'ever had' an alcoholic drink. Similar proportions reported having been 'really drunk' at least once. Approximately 50% of English young people who drank in the previous four weeks reported feeling drunk (58% of girls and 49% of boys). Around 40% of thirteen year olds and 55% of fifteen year olds in Scotland reported at least one from a list of negative consequences associated with alcohol intoxication, the most commonly reported being 'having an argument' and 'vomiting'. Self-reported 'drunkenness' appears to be more common among Scottish young people. The extent or severity of drunkenness may also be relevant as the proportion of Scottish young people reporting being 'really drunk' was similar to English young people who reported 'feeling drunk'. The experience of drunkenness increases with age, and heavier drinking among young people is commonly associated with use of tobacco and other drugs.

In Scotland between 2006 and 2008 there was a reduction from 14% to 11% of thirteen year olds and from 36% to 31% of fifteen year olds who reported consuming alcohol in the previous week. In the same period in England there was a reduction in 11–15 year olds who reported drinking alcohol in the previous week, from 26% in 2006 to 18% in 2008 (NHS Information Centre, 2010). Whilst reported drinking in this age group is similar to that recorded in 1990, peaks of 20% and 47% (thirteen and fifteen year olds respectively) were recorded in 1996 peaking again in 2002 at 23% and 46% for thirteen and fifteen year olds respectively (SALSUS, 2008;

ISD, 2011). The changes in reported drinking in young people, in both countries, mirrored the reported consumption of the general adult population during the same period, with a higher proportion of Scottish young people admitting to consumption in the previous week.

More than half of thirteen year olds and less than 40% of fifteen year old Scottish young people and 48% of 11–15 year olds in England who reported that they had ever had a drink indicated that they had never actually bought alcohol. Provision by, or purchasing alcohol from, friends and relatives appears to be the most consistent and increasing source of alcohol as the percentage of those reporting purchase directly from off-licence and on-licence premises has significantly decreased since the early 1990s. Whilst this trend may reflect increased vigilance on so-called 'underage drinking' on the part of licence holders (both on- and off-licence), it also reflects the general population shift towards purchasing from off-licence premises (including supermarkets) at lower prices and a permissive attitude to the provision of alcohol to younger people. The role of alcohol advertising and sponsorship also contributes to a positive attitude towards alcohol among younger people, which is predictive of subsequent drinking (Babor *et al.*, 2003). The case study illustrates some of these themes.

CASE STUDY — TOO MUCH TOO YOUNG

Janice, aged fourteen, first tasted an alcoholic drink when she was twelve and thought that it was disgusting. She occasionally has small diluted alcoholic drinks on special occasions, with a family meal. She arranged to go out with her friends after having her dinner with her family, and met up with a large crowd of twenty fellow school students, some of whom she knew. Older youths freely passed around two litre bottles of 'lemonade'. As the crowd grew more gregarious neighbours called the police. As the police arrived the young people fled, with the exception of Janice, who was unconscious. Police took her to accident and emergency, where she remained until her parents arrived to take her home. She was not charged with any offence.

Other than a nasty hangover she was unharmed. She has no recollection of the gathering after a couple of hours and whilst she thinks she was drinking a vodka concoction, amongst other drinks, has no idea how much she consumed. She has no recollection of being in hospital.

Janice is embarrassed, contrite towards her parent and upset that her friends did not look after her. She was provided with alcohol information leaflets, but refused to read them, having had similar information at school.

Implications

Janice did at least have meal before going out and was not drinking on an empty stomach. The importance of joining in with her peers and the importance of getting drunk fits with young peoples' common attitudes and behaviour in relation to drinking. Drinking outdoors is common. Adolescents 12–14 years old tend to drink a wide variety of beverages including alcopops (ready to drink) and as they get older they narrow their drinking repertoire in favour of more 'adult' drinks. Janice appears to have been oblivious to her alcohol consumption. She put herself in a very vulnerable situation on the basis of her apparent high level of intoxication and inability to look after herself.

Janice's contact with the police — called to deal with a disturbance or someone who is drunk and incapable — is not unusual. The same may be said for her time spent at accident and emergency. Cleary, there are cost implications associated with police time as well as NHS staff and resources in dealing with the effects of drunkenness. While alcohol information or education is an important part of citizenship there is little evidence of it as a preventive strategy to delay starting drinking or reduce alcohol consumption. The opposing messages from friends and media are more powerful.

Social and cultural influences

Socio-economic class

DOH (1998), an independent inquiry on health inequalities, notes a clear relationship between socio-economic class and morbidity and mortality. Death rates were noted to be significantly higher among unskilled men and those from professional households. Over a lengthy period GHS has shown little difference in the weekly consumption of alcohol between manual and non-manual households. Any difference identified tended to be in non-manual households, where higher consumption was associated with higher disposable income. Similar conclusions, with a strong emphasis on the role of alcohol drugs and violence, are reached by the ministerial task force on health inequalities (Scottish Government, 2008b).

Robinson *et al.* (2011) report that in 2009 in the UK average weekly alcohol consumption was highest, at 13.5 units, in the professional/ managerial group, with 77% of men and 65% of women having had an alcoholic drink in the last seven days; it was lowest, at 10.7 units, among those in manual households, where 59% of men and 44% of women had had an alcoholic drink in the previous seven days. This is a consistent finding for both men and women; however, the difference is greater when professional women are compared to women in manual households where their weekly consumption is 9.7 units and 6.6 units per week, respectively.

Women in professional/managerial households were twice as likely to drink more than three units in any one day by comparison to women from manual households. They were also twice as likely to have drunk heavily on at least one occasion in the previous week. A similar but smaller distinction was apparent when comparing men from professional and manual households. Bromley and Shelton (2010) suggest that levels of deprivation alone do not explain differences in health outcomes between the regions and nations of the UK. This issue will be developed further in Chapter 2.

Ethnicity

In the UK survey (NHS Information Centre, 2010), respondents from Pakistani or Bangladeshi origin in the UK were unlikely to have had a drink in the previous week, 5% and 4% respectively, compared to 68% among those who described themselves as 'white British'. Such low levels of alcohol consumption in a large ethnic community could serve to reduce the average alcohol consumption in particular geographical areas.

Looking at ethnicity on the basis of religious affiliation presents a contrasting picture. Cochrane and Bal (1990) investigated the alcohol consumption of Sikh, Hindu, Muslim and white English males in the West Midlands. Alcohol consumption levels and patterns of drinking among males from the different ethnic groups were quite different, as were the consequences of drinking. In Muslim culture, where alcohol consumption was expressly forbidden, those very few males who did consume alcohol were very heavy consumers and deviant from their cultural and religious norms. The weekly consumption of alcohol by the Sikh and white English males was very similar. However, when problems were considered the Sikhs reported family tensions in relation to their drinking while the white English males reported much higher levels of 'police trouble'. This reflects the regular drinking of

Sikh males in comparison to the binge-style drinking of the white English males and the legal consequences which can ensue as well as the different cultural influences brought to bear on alcohol consumption and related conduct.

Conclusions

Per capita alcohol consumption has risen substantially in recent decades, reaching a peak in the middle of the first decade of the twenty-first century, followed by modest decline. Despite this reduction, consumption, relative to preceding decades, is high. Consumption is sensitive to the price of alcohol and in relation to overall consumer expenditure, so cheaper alcohol has resulted in increased consumption. However, recent economic changes will have contributed to the downturn in the period from 2008, making alcohol relatively more expensive.

Alcohol consumption is difficult to measure, given the range of strength in which alcoholic beverages are available. There is a significant gap apparent between sales data and the responses given in population surveys. Despite this there are important and consistent findings, noting increases and decreases in consumption over time. Surveys present a broadly consistent picture of declining alcohol consumption in the early twenty-first century, from 2006 to 2009. There has been a significant shift in sales from the on-trade licensed premises to off-trade or off-licence premises, including supermarkets, where price per unit of alcohol is significantly cheaper, perhaps altering drinking patterns and consequences.

Per capita alcohol consumption, based on sales data and self-reports of drinking, is higher in Scotland compared with the rest of the UK. Young people in Scotland more commonly report instances of having been 'very drunk' than in England. Scottish adults report higher levels of alcohol consumption including a greater likelihood of drinking in excess of recommended limits. Proportionately, both men and women in Scotland are more likely to drink in excess of recommended limits for both harmful and hazardous drinking than in England and Wales.

In addition to per capita consumption of alcohol, attention must also be paid to drinking patterns, some of which may be protective, others less so. Drinking patterns relate to the number of drinking days per week and the rate of consumption, both of which may be influenced by cultural norms, including beliefs about the meaning of drinking. As far as social background is concerned those with the highest income have the highest average consumption, partake in more drinking occasions and are more likely to consume over the recommended limits. Whilst consumption may be greater for those who are better off, negative alcohol-related consequences, including health, affect the less well-off much more despite their more modest average consumption.

Where there is a similarity in consumption levels between different ethnic groups (e.g. Hindu and English white males), the reported social consequences of drinking are quite different. Binge drinking and the antisocial behaviour and health consequences associated with this pattern of drinking are major sources of public concern across the UK, though this pattern of drinking appears to be more prevalent in Scotland.

On the basis of consumption measures alone it would be expected that Scotland would have higher levels of alcohol-related problems than other countries in the UK. The next chapter will consider the wide-ranging health and social consequences associated with alcohol consumption and will point out connections between per capita consumption and the prevalence of consequences, underpinned by the influences of deprivation.

CHAPTER 2

Alcohol: Health and Social Consequences

> There is a definite relationship between the consumption of alcoholic liquors and the incidence of alcoholic mortality. (Wilson, 1940, p. 307)

> WHO European Region has the highest proportion of total ill-health and premature death due to alcohol in the world, with a very close relationship between a country's total per capita alcohol consumption and its prevalence of alcohol-related harm and alcohol dependence. (WHO, 2010)

Alcohol contributes to 4% of the global 'burden of disease', which is as much death and disability globally as that associated with tobacco and hypertension (Room *et al.*, 2005). The burden may be considered higher still in those counties where both consumption and consequences are higher than the global average. This is most notable among the European nations (Rehm *et al.*, 2010), including Scotland.

Alcohol consumption in the UK — and Scotland in particular — is high and has had an impact on many aspects of life. Public concern, in the last decade, has focused mainly on binge drinking, by younger people and associated public disorder. This chapter will consider the costs associated with, and impact of alcohol on, health, offending and the family. The relationship between alcohol and health, including alcohol dependence, will be outlined. Deprivation and health inequality will be considered as a contributory to alcohol-related consequences and the contribution of alcohol to the 'Scottish or Glasgow Effect' on health outcomes will be explored.

Costs

The Department of Health (DOH) estimates the costs to the NHS for England and Wales at around £2.7 billion a year and alcohol-related admissions account for 7% of the total admissions to the NHS (NHS Information Centre, 2010). In Scotland the alcohol-related cost of healthcare in 2007, including primary care, community-based and hospital care was estimated to be around £269 million. Most of these costs are attributable to alcohol-related hospital admissions (psychiatric and non-psychiatric) accounting for 7.5% of the total societal costs of alcohol-related consequences in Scotland.

Scottish Government estimates the cost of alcohol-related crime, for 2007, at between £463 million and £992 million (mid-point £727 million), accounting for 20% of the total overall cost of alcohol misuse. Alcohol is implicated in a wide range of offences, some of which are alcohol specific (e.g. drink driving), while the majority are alcohol related (e.g. assault vandalism). Three-quarters of the costs associated with alcohol and offending result from costs as a consequence of the crimes, while one-fifth is attributed to the costs of the criminal justice system (police, courts, probation services and prison).

Social care costs associated with alcohol in Scotland amounted to between £114 million and £347 million (mid-point £230 million) in 2007. The majority of these costs are derived from social care relating to children and families, care homes, the Children's Hearing System and criminal justice social work (Beale *et al.*, 2009).

The relationships between alcohol and health
Safer drinking?

Alcohol consumption, in moderation, is generally promoted as a healthy activity; however, it is difficult to define. Drinking less than the government-recommended limits of fourteen units per week for women and twenty-one units per week for men is associated with reduced risk of alcohol-related health and social consequences and stands as a definition of harm-free or safer drinking. However, reduced risk does not imply that there will be no risk of alcohol-related consequences, as in some instances any alcohol consumption is risky: for example, driving, operating machinery. Low levels of alcohol consumption are associated with a reduction in the risk of cardiovascular heart disease, in men aged over forty, and women who are postmenopausal, where the 'benefit' of alcohol can largely be gained by drinking as little as one unit per day on a regular basis. No additional health benefits result from consumption above two units a day. Studies of cancers indicate that there is no safe limit for alcohol consumption below which the risk of cancer is avoided, though increased prevalence is associated with drinking in excess of recommended limits (Schutze, 2011). A low level of consumption, which may be beneficial in preventing one particular disease (cardiovascular disease) will not necessarily prevent the occurrence of another (alcohol-related cancers).

Alcohol, causality and health

Many acute and chronic diseases, and injuries, are affected by alcohol consumption and drinking patterns. Increased consumption is associated with increased risk. Alcohol is causally related to more than sixty medical conditions (Room et al., 2005). Where alcohol is 'wholly attributable', it makes a 100% contribution to conditions that are listed in international disease classifications (WHO, 1992). This implies that the condition would not occur if alcohol was not consumed. Where alcohol is 'partly attributable', then alcohol is one of a number of influences. The proportionate contribution of alcohol may vary from one disease to another, or vary for the same disease when women and men are compared. Diseases where alcohol has a causal influence are outlined below:

Alcohol and its causal impact on major health consequences

Wholly attributable

Tuberculosis

Diabetes

Alcoholic liver disease, including cirrhosis of the liver

Alcohol use disorders

Alcoholic polyneuropathy, myopathy ,cardiomyopathy, gastritis and pancreatitis

Alcohol-related degeneration of the nervous system (alcohol related brain damage, includingWenicke's Korsakoff's syndrome)

Intentional and accidental poisoning by alcohol

Epilepsy

Unipolar depressive disorders

Lower respiratory infections (pneumonia)

Pre-term birth complications and foetal alcohol syndrome (FAS)

Partly or proportionately attributable

Cancers: mouth, nasopharynx, other pharynx and oropharynx, oesophageal cancer, colon and rectum cancer, liver cancer, breast cancer, in women

Hypertensive heart disease, ischaemic heart disease (IHD), ischaemic and haemorrhagic stroke, conduction disorders and other dysrhythmias

Injuries: road traffic accidents, fire injuries, assaults, accidents and intentional self-harm

Psoriasis, epilepsy, spontaneous abortion

Source: Rehm et al., 2010; Information Services Division, 2011

Non-communicable disease

> Together with smoking, diet and physical inactivity, con-
> sumption of alcohol is among the four most important risk
> factors for non-communicable disease (NCDs). Alcohol
> consumption, especially heavy consumption, impacts on
> cancer, liver cirrhosis and stroke. (Room *et al.*, 2011, p. 1547)

Binge drinking is associated with increased risk for some diseases and many injuries (Rehm *et al.*, 2010; Gmel *et al.*, 2011). In a study comparing 10,000 male drinkers from France and Northern Ireland, over a ten-year period, 9% of middle-aged males were found to be binge drinkers, most commonly at weekends, compared to 0.5% in France. Around 75% of French men drank daily, but less per drinking session, compared to 12% of men from Northern Ireland. Binge drinkers had almost twice the risk of heart attack or death from heart disease, when compared with regular drinkers.

In a study on the burden of cancer attributed to both current and former drinkers in eight European countries, including the UK, Schutze *et al.* (2011) conclude that there was a causal link between alcohol consumption in 10% of cancers in males and 3% in females, in Europe, with a substantial proportion associated with consumption at levels greater than the recommended limits (Table 2.1). In the UK alcohol is implicated in 8% of cancer cases in males and 3% in females. Compared to Europe the prevalence in the UK is slightly lower for men and the same for women. The proportion of cancers attributable to alcohol increases markedly — both in Europe and the UK — when cancers with a causal relationship are considered (i.e. wholly attributable), being 32% and 5% in men and women respectively.

Table 2.1: Proportion of cancer cases (in %) attributable to alcohol use in males and females aged 15+: UK and Europe.

Cancer	UK		Europe	
	Men (%)	Women (%)	Men (%)	Women (%)
Total cancer	8	3	10	3
Alcohol 'causal' cancers				
Upper aero-digestive tract*	45	30	44	25
Colorectum	14	5	17	4
Liver	33	13	33	18
Breast		5		5

* Upper aero-digestive tract cancers: oral cavity, pharynx, larynx, oesophagus: Source: Schutze *et al.*, 2011

Table 2.1 indicates that, with the exception of breast cancer, alcohol-attributed cancers are higher amongst men than women. The incidence of alcohol-attributable cancer was highest in relation to the upper aero-digestive tract, where the proportion was slightly higher in the UK compared to Europe. Cancer of the liver was the same between men and lower for women in UK, when compared to Europe.

Among injecting drug users hazardous and harmful alcohol consumption presents serious risks to the long-term recipient of methadone and other opioid-substitute medication. Alcohol is commonly reported as one of the drugs present when a drug-related death is recorded and more than 70% of regular drug injectors are hepatitis C positive. Continued hazardous alcohol consumption may potentially result in poor prognosis for hepatitis C and increase demand for liver transplant.

Alcohol dependence

Alcohol dependence, sometimes referred to as alcohol addiction, is defined in the International Classification of Mental and Behavioural Disorders (ICD-10) as 'a cluster of physiological, behavioural and cognitive phenomena in which the use of a substance or class of substances takes on a much higher priority for a given individual than other behaviours' (WHO, 1992).

A diagnosis of alcohol dependence is commonly made if three or more of the following criteria have been evidenced in the previous year:

- a strong desire or compulsion to consume: sometimes described as 'craving';
- difficulty in controlling consumption: may be associated with craving but also related to the difficulty in keeping to a limit on a drinking occasion;
- physiological withdrawal state: commonly sweats, nausea, tremor and more seriously seizures and dementia tremens;
- evidence of tolerance: need to consume increasing amounts in order to achieve desired effect;
- progressive neglect of social and other activities: salience of drinking over family, employment and other roles.

In England the prevalence of alcohol dependence was estimated to be 3.6% (6% men and 2% women) or around 1.1 million people. Regional variation was noted for the prevalence of alcohol dependence in East Midlands (1.6%) and in the North-east and Yorkshire and Humber (5.2%) (Drummond *et al.*, 2005). In Scotland, based on 2006 data, it is estimated that alcohol dependence is around 6% (SMACAP, 2011). The higher prevalence rate overall for alcohol dependence in Scotland is largely accounted for by the higher prevalence of alcohol dependence in women (Drummond *et al.*, 2009).

Among illicit drug users in England and Wales, of the 1,075 individuals entering treatment for drug problems a significant proportion were drinking harmfully, in addition to illicit drug use (Gossop *et al.*, 2003). Over the follow-up period of five years, significant reductions in illicit drug use and associated offending were noted, but no similar reduction in alcohol consumption. In a community drug service study in Scotland, O'Rawe (2006) reports harmful levels of alcohol consumption in a cohort of service users prescribed maintenance methadone, including around 20% who had been in contact with specialist alcohol services.

Co-morbidity, or dual diagnosis, refers to the co-occurrence of harmful drinking, including dependence, and mental health problems (mental illness) in an individual at a particular point in their life. In community surveys Jenkins *et al.* (1997) report a strong correlation between mental health symptoms and alcohol use; that is, as mental health symptoms increase so does substance use. There are a number of different ways in which the relationships between alcohol and mental illness can be explained, which depend on the level of alcohol consumption and the specific mental health condition. A study of the prevalence of co-morbidity found that in specialist alcohol services the prevalence of mental health conditions was significant: affective and anxiety disorders 81%, personality disorders 53%, schizophrenia 3%. In community and mental health services, 44% of service users reported a problem with alcohol or illicit drugs in the previous year (Weaver *et al.*, 2003). Similarly, high levels of prevalence of co-morbidity are also noted in both prison and homeless populations (Scottish Executive, 2003b).

Health harm: Scotland

This section will outline the impact of alcohol on health services.

Primary care

Primary care refers to GP and health centres where the largest proportion of the population have contact with health services. Between 2004/5 and 2008/9 there was a reduction of around 7% from 115,335 to 107,414 contacts, where alcohol was a wholly attributable cause. In 2008/9 this translated to between 38,000 and 50,000 patients, who on average consulted on slightly more than two occasions. Those most deprived were around 4.5 times more likely to have such a health contact compared to those least deprived (ISD, 2011). This underestimates the real burden on primary care services as records of contacts where alcohol is 'partly attributable' are not included.

Emergency hospital admissions

Alcohol accounted for 92% of emergency admissions in 2009/10. This consists of alcohol-related accidents (trauma, assaults) and emergency admissions for alcohol-related conditions. NHSScotland (NHS Quality Improvement Scotland, 2005) published clinical indicators for alcohol-related emergency hospital admissions between 1996/7 and 2003/4. Table 2.2 lists the most common alcohol-related emergency admissions. Substantial increases in rates (per 10,000 of the population) of emergency admissions are apparent over the period, for both men and women: for example, a 100% increase in the rate of emergency admissions for chronic liver disease among women; and a 96% increase in the rate of emergency admission for chronic pancreatitis among men. Increased alcohol-related emergency admissions during this period also reflected the increase in both alcohol sales and reported consumption during the same period. The percentage increase in emergency admissions for these conditions, irrespective of gender, is striking. As with other alcohol-related consequences admissions increase significantly among those who are most deprived. Those most deprived are seven times more likely to be admitted as an emergency for acute alcohol intoxication, six times more likely to be admitted as an emergency for liver disease and eight times more likely to be admitted as an emergency for chronic pancreatitis, whether male or female.

Table 2.2: Emergency admission rates for alcohol-related conditions 1996/7 to 2003/4

Alcohol-related condition	Increase (%) in rate per 10,000	Deprivation: Most compared to least deprived
Acute intoxication males females	 40% 30%	7 fold increase in admission (male and female)
Liver disease males females	 71% 83%	6+ fold increase in admission (male and female)
Chronic liver disease males females	 92% 100%	2.7 fold increase in admission (male and female)
Chronic pancreatitis males females	 96% 55%	8 fold increase in admission (male and female)
Oesophageal varices males females	 50% 33%	3 fold increase in admission (male and female)

Source: www.nhshealthquality.org

Alcohol-related hospital discharges

Alcohol-related discharges refer to general acute in-patient and day case discharges, excluding obstetric and psychiatric hospitals. In Scotland, from 2005/6 to 2009/10 there was a 2% increase in alcohol-related discharges from general acute hospitals, reaching a peak of 43,000 in 2007/8, whilst there was a reduction from 42,000 to 39,278 between 2008/9 and 2009/10. Alcohol-related discharges reflected the following breakdown in 2009: approximately 72%

'mental and behavioural disorders due to alcohol use' and approximately 17% alcoholic liver disease (one-quarter of which are cirrhosis of the liver). During this period discharges increased in the 20–44 age range whilst falling in both younger and older age groups. Discharges in 2009/10 involved a total of 26,257 patients with an alcohol-related diagnosis, meaning that these patients tended to be hospitalised on more than one occasion, in particular those in the 35–59 age group. The highest rate of alcohol-related discharge was in Greater Glasgow and Clyde health board area. Alcohol-related discharges were 7.5 times greater for the most deprived areas in comparison to the most affluent areas (ISD, 2011).

In Scotland over the five-year period 2004/5 and 2008/9, alcohol-related discharges from psychiatric hospitals decreased by around 5% (4,392 to 4,177), with alcohol dependence being recorded in 69% of discharges (3,000 to 2,926). These figures include both in-patient and out-patient discharges. The rate of discharge from deprived areas was nine times that of more affluent areas (ISD, 2011). Local variation reflects the range of specialist alcohol services operating in rural and urban areas, including those delivered by local authority social services and non-statutory bodies.

Alcohol-related deaths

Alcohol-related deaths in the UK refer to the underlying cause of death, namely the condition that initiated events leading to death. Instances where alcohol is contributory, but not recorded as the underlying cause, are excluded. This measure substantially underestimates the impact of alcohol on mortality. However, a broader definition includes 'any mention' of alcohol on a death certificate. When wholly attributable and partly attributable conditions are included in estimating the impact of alcohol and morbidity the picture changes significantly. The inclusion of 'any mention' of alcohol on a death certificate virtually doubles alcohol-related deaths.

In Scotland in 2003 it was estimated that there were 2,882 deaths from 'any mention' of alcohol attributable conditions, representing 5% of deaths in that year. In the sixteen- to twenty-four-year-old males, 17.5% of all deaths were attributable to alcohol. In this age group and those generally below the age of thirty-five the acute consequences of intoxication, involving intentional self-harm and traffic accidents were the main cause of death. By contrast, those over the age of thirty-five were more commonly affected by the chronic consequences of their alcohol consumption. In 2009 more than two-thirds of the alcohol-related deaths were of people over fifty years of age, the same for both men and women. The death rate for men, of all ages, where alcohol is an underlying cause, is double that of women (ISD, 2011).

In Scotland between 2005 and 2009 there were fluctuations in the number of cases where alcohol was an underlying cause of death. Overall, there was a 15% reduction, consisting of 18% reduction among men and 10% reduction in women. With regard to deprivation, rates of alcohol-related deaths ranged from 7.8 times greater (2008) to 6.3 times greater (2009) for the most deprived compared to the least deprived. In 2007 the alcohol-related mortality rate was almost double in Scotland compared to England and Wales (Gartner, 2009).

In Scotland in 2009 53,856 deaths were recorded and 1,282 (2.4%) were instances where alcohol was the underlying cause, representing a 10% reduction on the previous year. By considering 'any cause' the deaths attributable to alcohol rise to approximately 2,560. Drug-related deaths in the same year exceeded 500 and alcohol was a significant contributory factor.

Deprivation

Health inequalities are an outcome of deprivation and poverty (Acheson, 1998; Scottish Government, 2008b). Virtually every health measure associated with alcohol demonstrates a poorer outcome for those most deprived compared with the most affluent. Poor alcohol-related health markers and outcomes are not necessarily due to those less well-off consuming more alcohol than those more affluent. The reverse is the case. Deprivation explains health inequalities, and differences in health outcomes between Scotland and the rest of the UK, but not completely.

THE 'SCOTTISH/GLASGOW EFFECT'

Deprivation is a fundamental determinant of health. The so-called 'Glasgow effect' refers to the higher levels of mortality and morbidity experienced in the deprived postindustrial region of west central Scotland, with Glasgow at its centre, which exceeds that which may be explained by deprivation alone (Hanlon *et al.*, 2006; McCartney *et al.* 2011; Bromley and Shelton, 2010). These measures are so significant that they skew the overall picture of Scotland's health. The 'Glasgow effect' reflects a slower rate of health improvement in the city compared to the rest of the UK, a phenomenon that may date from the early 1980s. A similar effect has also been reported in both Wales and north-east England (Bromley and Shelton, 2010).

Glasgow has been compared to Manchester and Liverpool, cities with almost identical deprivation profiles. Gray (2007) notes that alcohol consumption was greater in Glasgow than the rest of Scotland. For the period 2003–7, standardised all-cause mortality ratio (SMR) comparisons demonstrated that in Glasgow there were 30% more premature deaths, with all deaths 15% higher than would be expected given the similarity in deprivation profile between the three cities. It is estimated that in the study period that there were 4,500 'excess' deaths in Glasgow, of which 46% occurred in those under the age of sixty-five. In more deprived areas of the city, premature deaths tended to be higher, particularly among males, and around half of these 'excess' deaths in those under the age of sixty-five were directly attributable to alcohol (32%) and drugs (17%) (Hanlon *et al.*, 2006).

Alcohol-related causes of death were 2.3 times greater for Glasgow compared to Liverpool and Manchester and similarly 2.5 times greater for drug-related deaths (in which alcohol is also implicated).

Whilst there are many theories that seek to explain these phenomena there is a general acceptance that substance use, and alcohol in particular, play a significant part in understanding the 'Glasgow effect' (McCartney *et al.*, 2011).

'Given the high mortality rates for alcohol, drugs and lung cancer seen in Glasgow this perhaps suggests an extreme behavioural risk profile among some elements of the Glasgow population, which is not identified from routine health surveys and prevalence data' (GCPH, 2010, p. 6).

Alcohol and offending
The relationships between alcohol and offending
Alcohol is not criminogenic, that is, it does not cause crime. If it did cause crime then all alcohol consumers would offend. Clearly they do not. Alcohol and crime appear to be associated at a population level. However, there are a number of important associations and many offenders, and victims, have alcohol in their blood at the time of the offence. A direct link between alcohol and crime implies that the offence would not have occurred in the absence of alcohol. Home Office (2003) defines alcohol-related crime as: 'Instances of crime

and disorder that occurred and/or occurred at that level of serious-
ness because alcohol consumption was a contributory factor.'

Indirect associations may affect crime in the following ways:

- encouraging crime in order to access or afford alcohol;
- alcohol problems produce a home environment conducive to
  crime and antisocial behaviour;
- alcohol facilitates crime in individuals with low impulse
  control;
- triggers or facilitates aggression;
- has a negative impact on inhibition judgement and
  decision-making;
- some offences may be recorded because the offender is too
  drunk to escape;
- drunks may be easily victimised;
- creates a scapegoat or excuse for bad behaviour, however
  serious.

As alcohol is widely available in the UK alcohol-related offending
is concerned with conduct 'under the influence' and requires an
understanding of individual and environmental or contextual factors. By contrast, in the case of illicit drugs prohibition dictates that
the main offences relate to possession and supply of drugs.

Drinking

In certain locations drinking or possession of alcohol is an offence.
Possession of alcohol is banned by law in sports grounds in Scotland. Similarly, since 1993, local authorities have had the power to
introduce by-laws which ban drinking alcohol in particular 'designated places' such as town and city centres. Whilst there has been a
three-fold increase between 2000/1 and 2009/10 in recorded offences
of drinking in designated places, the rise is primarily due to the
gradual uptake and implementation of such by-laws across Scotland in that period. Similar bans on drinking in public places have
emerged across the UK, a measure designed to limit alcohol-fuelled
public disorder. According to Robert Hamilton, chief superinten-
dent, Strathclyde Police: 'In Strathclyde our gangs are primarily
involved in territorial and recreational violence fuelled by alcohol'
(*Herald*, 12 August 2011).

Drunkenness

> Not drunk is he who from the floor
> Can rise alone and still drink more
> But drunk is They who prostrate lies
> Without the power to drink or rise
> (Thomas Love Peacock 1785–1866)

It has been suggested that drunkenness in the UK is 'the time-honoured cause for concern about alcohol' (Raistrick *et al.*, 1999, p. 4). Drunkenness can be a significant influence on a wide range of offending behaviour (e.g. breach of the peace, crimes of violence), which is not formally recorded as alcohol-related offences. 'Drunk and incapable' refers to persons who are intoxicated to such a level that it is impossible for them to look after themselves. As a result these individuals are vulnerable and at risk of harm to themselves and/or others. This covers a diverse group of individuals: some of whom are identified by the police on one occasion and never reappear; binge drinkers or regular heavy drinkers who appear on more than one occasion; and 'chronic recidivists' who are identified regularly and are commonly alcohol dependent.

In 2006/7, in Scotland, the cost of holding drunk and incapable individuals in police cells was £2.12 million. The impact on health services of this particular group in the same period was between £0.7 million and £1.95 million where between 7,500 and 21,000 attended accident and emergency services at a cost of £93 per hospital visit with a further cost of £0.7 million for acute hospital beds at a cost of £483 per day. As a consequence of these costs there is a need for a service response to drunk and incapable individuals (Griesbach *et al.*, 2009).

In prison populations around 50% of prisoners (male and female) indicate that they were drunk at the time of the offence. There is a marked difference where 77% of young offenders (under twenty-one years of age) compared to 44% of adult offenders admit to being drunk at the time of the offence. Screening the prison population in 2007 and 2009 resulted in just under half of the prison population having an alcohol problem.

Violence and homicide

In more than 60% of reported violent crimes the victim believed that their attacker was under the influence of alcohol (ISD, 2011). This view was more common among male than female victims, as well as younger compared with older victims. Almost half of younger victims were under the influence of alcohol at the time of their attack.

For homicide cases in Scotland in 2009/10 being under the influence of alcohol or drugs was known for 65% of the accused: 33% of the accused were under the influence of alcohol; while 12% were under the influence of both alcohol and drugs. The percentage of those accused of homicides, who were under the influence of alcohol or drugs, has fluctuated between 36% and 56% in the period 2005/6 and 2009/10.

MURDER IN PRIVATE

Strathclyde police report a 73% increase in murders comparing April to November 2010 with the same period in 2009, which represents a 4.4% increase on the average for the previous five years. Such an increase contradicts the significant downward trends in attempted murder (29%), serious assaults (26%) and common assaults (9%).

A conclusion reached by the police force is that, of forty recorded homicides in April to November 2010, 60% are 'inside jobs'. The murders increase in places most difficult to police: the home or private place, commonly drinking parties. According to David Leask, the key factors involved appear to be:

○ Cheap alcohol bought from off-licences or supermarkets compared to the more expensive licensed premises.

○ Private drinking parties take place out-with the gaze of the police, who react robustly to street disorder and violence or publicans who would be duty bound to respond to drunkenness.

○ Drinking and drink-fuelled violence in private are more dangerous than in a pub or public place, where there are greater controls on behaviour and a greater likelihood of emergency services being called by a sober individual.

○ At a heavy drinking party, drunken participants do not react to control the risky behaviour of others and perhaps fail to act quickly enough when violence occurs. Consequently 70% of all murder victims attacked in private settings die at the scene. The opposite is the case for those hurt in public and they tend to lose their lives in hospital, whereby a majority survive (*Sunday Herald*, 2010).

Drink driving: Law and health

The Road Traffic Act 1967 introduced the drink driving legal limit of 80mg alcohol per 100ml blood (or 35mg alcohol per 100ml breath), and in its first seven years 5,000 deaths and 200,000 crashes were prevented (Dunbar, 1992). Alcohol affects driving skills (e.g. co-ordination, judgement, risk awareness) at low levels of consumption, certainly well below the legal limit in the UK, which is higher than in several other European countries. Individual differences, gender, weight, recent food consumption, rate and pattern of drinking all contribute to blood alcohol/breath measures.

Prevalence of drinking and driving (any alcohol) has decreased since 2001 both in terms of ever having driven after drinking (from 55% to 43%, 2001–7) and in having done so in the previous year (down from 37% to 35%, 2001–7) (Collins *et al.*, 2008). Those convicted of drunk driving tend to be younger people, while persistent offenders are commonly harmful or problem drinkers.

Drunk-driving offences in Scotland have fluctuated between 2000/1 and 2009/10, the number of offences having declined by less than 20%. However, a 13% reduction is noted in drunk-driving offences between 2008/9 and 2009/10. The rate for drunk driving across Scottish police force areas varied significantly in 2009/10, with Lothian and Borders at sixteen offences and Northern at twenty-two offences per 10,000 population, reflecting both police practice and geography. With regard to road accidents involving injury 59% of motorists (11,000) were requested to take a breath test with 4% refusing, in 2009. Most positive breath tests occurred at the weekend and between 9pm and 3am. The annual average for drunk-driving accident casualties, between 1999 and 2003, was forty-six fatalities with 180 serious injuries, reducing to thirty fatalities and 130 serious injuries per annum between 2004 and 2008 (ISD, 2011). In a study of alcohol-affected drivers, older drivers, including those who drive as part of their job, had higher liver enzyme measures (gamma glutamyl transferase, GGT), a measure of harmful drinking, which was associated with traffic accidents but not blood alcohol concentrations or previous convictions (Dunbar, 1992).

OVER WHAT LIMIT?

Alan is eighty-four years old and has been driving since his teens, whilst working on farms and later in life as a lorry driver. He prides himself on his driving skills and his exploits as a 'real driver'. He has been widowed for ten years and is fiercely independent and enjoys a drink most days, sometimes with friends and family or on his own 'for company'. His family joke with him that it's about time he stopped driving, though they are increasingly concerned at his erratic driving and the potential for him to injure himself or others. He is adamant that he will stop driving as he will know when the time is right.

Alan reversed his car into a neighbour's car, causing substantial damage. The police were called and seeing Alan upset and unsteady on his feet decided to breathalyse him. He was just below the legal limit (60mg/100ml) and was taken to the police station, where he was treated very kindly, and retested. Again, he was below the legal limit. He was mystified by this incident and admitted that his memory of the event was hazy.

Some weeks later his GP, as part of a routine health screening, asked Alan about his alcohol consumption and also took a blood sample. Alan's blood sample showed a raised GGT. The GP, suspicious about Alan's alcohol consumption, was duty bound to report the matter to DVLA, and advised Allan to stop driving for six month, or until the blood test showed a result in the normal range.

Implications

Under what circumstances is it advisable for older people to stop driving? Alcohol affects judgement and reaction time at blood/breath alcohol measures significantly below the legal limit. Alan may drink less than he used to, which is consistent with many older people; however, he does drink regularly, both in company and alone. This combination is associated with drinking at hazardous levels, which, given his age, may have an impact on his driving skills. He has committed no offence.

GGT indicates hazardous or harmful consumption of alcohol. Whilst this is not an offence, the Driver Vehicle Licensing Authority (DVLA) issues guidance on substance-use issues which requires a GP to report such a finding and that the driver stops driving for six months' minimum with a view to demonstrating subsequently a reduction in GGT to within set norms. This may be viewed as a public health intervention and road accident prevention strategy, the DVLA's underlying assumption being that alcohol consumption at a level that raises GGT implies an increased likelihood of driving whilst under the influence of alcohol.

Scottish Government has pressured UK Government, proposing a reduction in the drink-driving legal limit to 50mg alcohol per 100ml blood. This would result in a drink driving conviction for Alan.

Family

The vast majority of survey respondents described in Chapter 1 are family members. Similarly, the consequences of alcohol consumption, whether concerned with health, offending or employment, happen to people who are members of a family. As a consequence, a significant number of family members are likely to be affected by the hazardous and harmful drinking of one or more family members.

Both New Zealand and Australia have strong cultural ties with the UK and a similar per capita consumption of alcohol. In a general population survey of 3,000 New Zealand residents, 80% of whom were European, it was found that there was a relationship between reduced quality of life, poorer health and contact with heavy drinkers. Nearly 30% of respondents reported having at least one heavy drinker in their life and 19% reported one. One in four of respondents indicated that the heavy drinker was a member of their household (Casswell *et al.*, 2011). Similarly in a survey of 2,600 adult Australians, 30% indicated that the drinking of someone close to them had negative effects and 11% were affected by such a person 'a lot'. The harms reported ranged from noise and fear to physical abuse, sexual coercion and social isolation (Laslett *et al.*, 2011). The implication is that heavy drinkers may have a significant negative impact on those around them. These findings are important as they raise the issue of the unmeasured cost of alcohol, particularly in families, as opposed to studies conducted on clinical or service-user populations. The impact on those living with a harmful/dependent drinker are demonstrated in a US study of healthcare needs and service use of the family members of people with alcohol or drug problems (Ray *et al.*, 2009). They were more likely to suffer trauma, depression and have their own substance-use problem. Consequently, they used health services more often and at greater cost compared to family members of people suffering from other chronic conditions, specifically diabetes and asthma.

Similarly, studies evaluating the impact of interventions targeted at the 'concerned significant other' consistently report that those who engage with Alanon (a mutual support group for the relatives of problem drinkers) experience marked reductions in what were clearly high levels of stress and mental ill-health, prior to service contact. Additionally, cognitive behavioural interventions also increased the likelihood of the 'drinker' engaging in treatment services (Barber and Crisp, 1995; Meyers and Miller, 2002). Similarly, studies of treatment outcome for alcohol dependence report a reduction in the stress levels of concerned significant others when problem drinking reduces or ceases (Copello and Orford, 2002; Orford *et al.*, 2005). According to a female partner of a dependent drinker:

> It's extremely stressful ... you just don't know from one minute to the next just how things are going to be. There's never any consistency. There's constant ups and downs ... like a roller coaster ... you're constantly in a state of tension. There's always tension or anxiety floating around you. (Orford *et al.*, 2005, p. 26)

The impact of excessive and dependent drinking on the family (however defined) is difficult to measure. Young peoples' drinking is influenced in the early stages by family members. Drinking patterns that are excessive or problematic are likely to provide young people with negative role models for drinking. Parental drinking patterns tend to be replicated by children later in life such that around two-thirds of treatment-seeking adults, who are dependent on alcohol, commonly report problem drinking in one or more parent. Alcohol problems and dependence appear to run in families (Scottish Executive, 2003a).

It is estimated that 65,000 Scottish children live in a household where a parent's drinking is problematic (Scottish Government, 2008c). Glasgow social services report that between 66% and 75% of child protection cases involve alcohol and drug issues. Research in Bermondsey (Forrester, 2000) reported that substance use was strongly associated with neglect and that such cases were twice as likely to result in formal care proceedings. A substantial proportion of children on the Child Protection Register are affected by substance use (Scottish Executive, 2006; Scottish Government 2008a, 2008c, 2010a). In the UK more than 60% of cases of domestic violence involve alcohol (Home Office, 2003). A connection between child abuse cases, domestic abuse and per capita consumption of alcohol in North America was reported by Wagenaar *et al.* (2009).

> Those who underestimate the power of alcohol misuse to dis-rupt parenting and child care, merely continue the inappro-priate acceptance of alcohol misuse, that for years has plagued child care systems. (Harbin and Murphy, 2000, p. 2)

Conclusions

Alcohol consumption contributes very significantly to poor health in Scotland. Alcohol-related consequences, whether associated with health offending or the family, are linked to per capita consump-tion. Measures of alcohol-related consequences tend to rise and fall mirroring alcohol sales data and self-reported alcohol consumption from surveys. Therefore, reductions in consumption in the UK as a whole are reflected in decrements in many alcohol-related con-sequences in Scotland between 2005 and 2009. Given the levels of hazardous and harmful drinking it is clear that the alcohol problem in Scotland, and the UK, is not simply a matter of alcohol depend-ence or 'alcoholism'.

In a UK context Scotland's alcohol consumption and health con-sequences are high, having reduced from a peak around the early part of the first decade in the twenty-first century. Virtually every aspect of healthcare is impacted by the effects of alcohol, ranging from emergency hospital admissions, chronic health consequences of alcohol use, both in primary care and general hospital settings and alcohol-related deaths. There is also a significant impact on psychi-atric services, most of which is attributable to alcohol dependence. Similar reductions are reflected in alcohol-related offending includ-ing drink driving and violent offences. Both alcohol-related health consequences and offending impact on families and communities. Furthermore, hazardous and harmful drinking have a direct effect on family functioning, including parenting.

Deprivation accounts for substantial differences in the impact of alcohol on those who are most deprived compared with the most affluent. Virtually every alcohol-related health indicator suggests that there is a greater impact on those who are less affluent. Health inequality is not restricted to substance use and means that those living in poorer circumstances experience greater health problems and in turn make less effective use of health and social services. Alcohol-related offending is associated with deprivation — drink driving being the exception.

Deprivation alone cannot account for the marked differences in health, which show Scotland to have significantly worse health outcomes compared with the rest of the UK. It is possible that the source of this health inequality rests in west central Scotland, having been entitled the 'Scottish/Glasgow effect'. The impact of substance use — cheap and available alcohol in particular — is a strong contributory factor.

Geographical variations exist, both in the UK and across Scotland, in measurement and records of alcohol-related consequences, whether health or social in nature, reflecting both the underlying prevalence in the community and health, policing and social care policies and practices. The social determinants of drinking and alcohol-related problems are a key element in understanding the bigger picture as opposed to an individually focused explanation of alcohol problems. Consequently, the evidence presented in the following chapter will consider the use of price as a mechanism for reducing alcohol consumption and related problems. One of the main determinants of alcohol problems — availability as influenced by the price of alcohol — will also be considered.

CHAPTER 3

Pricing Alcohol

> Changes in the overall consumption of alcoholic beverages
> have a bearing on the health of the people in any society.
> Alcohol control measures can be used to limit consump-
> tion: thus, control of alcohol availability becomes a public
> health issue. (Bruun *et al.*, 1975, pp. 12–13)

The pricing and taxation of alcohol are highly contentious areas
where the vested interests of the alcohol production and sale indus-
tries, individual liberty and state intervention, in the form of public
health, frequently collide. The regulation of price and taxation of
alcoholic beverages is widely used by governments to raise revenue
to support their need for resources to allocate to a variety of expen-
ditures. Additionally, in some countries, price control and taxation
have been used as a means of minimising alcohol-related harm. Generally, studies show that increases in price and tax on alcohol reduce
consumption and alcohol-related health and social consequences,
whilst cheaper alcohol results in increased consumption and greater
harm.

This chapter will consider the affordability of alcoholic beverages and the influence of price mechanisms on consumption. Policy
options for alcohol price regulation will be considered. Particular
attention will be paid to 'minimum unit pricing', a nuanced perspective, reflecting diversity in the population in terms of age, gender and
levels of consumption as well as preferences in drinking settings. The
current status of price control as a policy option in the UK as a whole
and in Scotland separately will be compared to earlier proposals to
control consumption and harm.

Affordability: drinking with your pocket

In the UK alcohol was 66% more affordable in 2009 compared to 1987. This has come about because, whilst the price of alcohol has increased more than the general retail prices of other commodities, household disposable income has increased substantially more in that period. During the same period, alcohol purchased from off-sales (off-licences, shops, supermarkets) has become considerably more affordable than on-trade (pubs, clubs, hotels, etc.). Beer in 2009 was 155% more affordable when bought from off-sales, compared with 39% more affordable from licensed premises. During the same period, spirits and wine, combined, became more affordable from licensed premises, 50% and 126% from off-licences respectively. Overall, alcohol is cheaper and more affordable still when purchased from off-sales.

In Scotland 80% of alcohol sold from off-sales is purchased at a cost of between twenty-five and fifty-five pence per unit of alcohol, with 75% of cider sold for less than forty pence per unit; in contrast, 8% of beer, 2% of light wine and 1% of spirits are sold at less than twenty-five pence per unit (ISD, 2011). In Edinburgh, 377 individuals with severe alcohol problems, in contact with a range of health services, including specialist treatment services, reported consuming an average of almost 200 units of alcohol in the previous week, with a maximum of up to 800 units per week (harmful drinking is in excess of fifty/thirty-five units per week for men and women). They reported buying alcohol at, on average, forty-three pence and as low as nine pence per unit. The lower the price the more the problem drinkers consumed, and cheapness was commonly offered as the reason for choice of beverage. Problem drinking subjects purchased alcohol more cheaply than the rest of the population and mainly from off-sales. As heavy consumers of the cheapest alcohol available, it is suggested that a small change in purchasing alcohol could have a relatively large impact on consumption (Black *et al.*, 2011).

Price mechanisms and consumption

Alcoholic beverages, like any other commodity, obey the economic rules of supply and demand. A limited supply and constant or increased demand will result in highly priced alcohol. The same high level of demand with unlimited supply, or decreased demand with a constant supply, will result in cheaper alcohol. The potential for price and taxation to be manipulated will in turn affect the relationships between supply and demand. Central to the use of price as a means of controlling purchase, and by implication consumption, is the concept of price elasticity of demand. This predicts the extent to which a given price increase or reduction will result in altered consumption and is defined as the percentage change in consumption resulting from 1% alteration in price. Price elasticity is important in developing a public health response whereby an increase in price will result in a decrease in consumption. By contrast, inelastic demand is useful for revenue-generation schemes as consumption remains unaltered whilst price and in turn revenues may be increased. The price elasticity of an alcoholic beverage is culturally driven and it cannot be assumed that the price elasticity of a beverage (e.g. beer) will be the same when two countries are compared. Different alcoholic beverages tend to have different elasticities, within the same country.

Table 3.1: Mean elasticity scores and reductions in consumption following 10% price increase

Beverage	Mean elasticity score	Price increase (%)	Reduction in consumption (%)	Number of supporting studies
Beer	-0.46	10	4.6	105
Wine	-0.69	10	6.9	93
Spirits	-0.80	10	8.0	103
Alcohol (overall)	-0.51	10	5.1	91
Heavy alcohol use	-0.28	10	2.8	10

Source: Wagenaar et al., 2009

Table 3.1 shows the mean elasticity of alcoholic beverages, and consequent reductions in per capita consumption, on the basis of a 10% increase in beverage price. Mean elasticity scores vary from one beverage to another. This score is aggregated for all alcoholic beverages. Alcoholic beverages are relatively 'inelastic' in that a 10% increase in price results in a lower percentage decrease in consumption, irrespective of beverage type. Price elasticity is lower for alcoholic beverages among heavy alcohol users, whose consumption is

affected by price changes, though to a lesser extent than the population as a whole. Larger reductions in consumption could be achieved
by increasing price further.

As the mean elasticity scores are based on a considerable number
of studies the price elasticity of specific beverages and alcohol would
not necessarily equate to any single country. Therefore, price elasticity for beverages in the UK, for example, will vary from those in the
table. Furthermore, within the UK there may be regional variations
in elasticity for particular beverages, which reflect a range of cultural
factors. Consequently:

> Estimates of tax and price effects also reflect particular
> meanings and uses of alcoholic beverages across diverse
> social and cultural environments, and tax and price policies
> probably interact with a whole web of individual, commu-
> nity and social influences on drinking behaviour. (Wage-
> naar *et al.*, 2009, p.189)

Many governments, on the basis of a variety of influences, are
reluctant to raise taxation on alcohol. The stability of these taxes
results in inflation eroding their value over time and, as a result, to a
decline in the real price of alcohol. However, Wagenaar *et al.* (2009)
conclude that the relatively inelastic demand for alcohol will result
in both reductions in consumption as well as the potential to sustain
or increase revenue:

> The responsiveness of alcohol consumption to its price
> affects not only the efficiency with which special alcohol
> taxes generate revenue but also the potential health ben-
> efits to be reaped from higher alcohol prices. (Babor *et al.*,
> 2003, p. 103)

In this sense the purpose of a public health approach and a revenue-
raising strategy are both served. The relative price of alcohol may
be influenced by factors other than public health or revenue-raising
strategies: for example, costs of housing, food and fuel.

Price change, altered consumption and harm
In a systematic review of 112 studies, highly significant relationships between alcohol tax or price measures, sales and self-reported

consumption were noted. Furthermore, price and tax also had a marked effect on heavy drinking, though this tended to be smaller than the effect on the overall alcohol consumption of the population as a whole, as can be seen in Table 3.1. Consequently, a large literature exists, which:

> demonstrates the statistically overwhelming evidence of effects of alcohol prices on drinking. Price affects drinking of all types of beverages, and across the population of drinkers from light drinkers to heavy drinkers ... at the most basic level, price interacts with income in affecting consumption. (Wagenaar *et al.*, 2009, pp. 187, 189)

These conclusions are supported by Chaloupka (2009) who considers that the findings provide a strong rationale for using increases in alcoholic beverage taxes to promote public health by reducing drinking. Similar sentiments are offered by Raistrick *et al.* (1999) in their summary of the evidence base for a UK alcohol policy and by Babor *et al.* (2003).

Chaloupka (2009) notes that in Alaska in both 1983 and 2002 alcoholic beverage tax increases reduced alcohol-related disease mortality significantly, including deaths from liver cirrhosis, acute alcohol poisoning, alcohol-related cancers, cardiovascular diseases. Furthermore, Chaloupka reports reductions in spouse abuse and physical child abuse and other violent behaviours as a result of increases in alcohol pricing and taxation. Geisbrecht *et al.* (2010) note the impact of consumption levels and the relationship with the 'second-hand effects of drinking' for populations and the resultant need for health priorities to focus more widely than the drinker.

In Finland, in 2004, a country where the high price of alcohol was a cornerstone of an effective public health strategy, taxes on alcohol were reduced. An association between tax cuts and an increase in the number of sudden deaths involving alcohol — a 17% increase on the previous year — was noted (Koski *et al.*, 2007). This reflected increases in alcohol consumption and alcohol-related consequences (Holder, 2007). Makela and Osterberg (2009) conclude, in a review of alcohol taxation in Finland, that the reductions in alcohol taxes in Finland in 2004 had the most significant effect on the poorer members of the population in terms of health damage due to reductions in alcohol prices and consequent increased consumption.

In 1980, the duty on alcohol was increased in the UK, resulting in an increase in the real cost of alcohol for the first time in several decades. During 1979–81 Kendell *et al.* (1983) conducted interviews with more than 400 'regular drinkers' in Scotland, before and after the price increase, giving an opportunity to assess the impact of the price change on levels of consumption as well as reported alcohol-related problems. It was concluded that the price increase resulted in marked decreases in alcohol consumption as well as levels of alcohol-related problems. Importantly, it also demonstrated that heavy drinkers reduced their consumption, too. In this instance, the price change was intended as a revenue-generating initiative, which yielded an unintended public health benefit.

Whilst the connection between price and availability, consumption and harm, is clear there is an absence of research in the UK ,and elsewhere, regarding the acceptability of price controls on alcohol. However, a study of family and friendship influences on young people's drinking habits in the UK indicated that the price of alcoholic drinks is more likely to limit alcohol consumption among young people than concerns about health or potential risks. It is suggested from focus groups that young people thought that the influence of the price of alcohol on consumption 'made sense' to young people (Sondhi and Turner, 2011). Those with commercial interests in the production and sale of alcohol tend to maintain that there is no connection between price, consumption and harm. According to D. Poley, chief executive of the Portman Group:

> The health lobby favours restrictive measures on pricing, availability, advertising, and marketing in the belief that this will reduce overall levels of consumption. Leaving aside some of the flaws in that assumption … rather than impose these blunt, ineffective measures that impact on the moderate majority … one should instead educate consumers into drinking responsibly. (Harkins and Poley, 2011, p. 21)

Pricing policy options

Taxation of alcoholic beverages to reduce consumption may be a clumsy process — commonly portrayed as using a sledgehammer to crack a nut — by the alcohol production and sales industry. Taxation increases may not result in a price increase for the consumer whereby retailers, including supermarkets, absorb the cost. Furthermore, taxation applied to alcoholic beverages bears little relation to alcohol content, in units, and potential harm and by contrast has evolved piecemeal for a variety of historical reasons (Donaldson and Rutter, 2011). Internationally, there is diversity in the policy approaches, which have been proposed, implemented or modelled in relation to alcohol price regulation. These include the following.

Inflation-linked taxation

The price of alcohol is linked to the rate of inflation. The cost of alcohol remains stable relative to other commodities, and as a result consumption is regulated. Failure to link beverage alcohol price to inflation tends to result in cheaper alcohol, increased consumption and resultant problems, as has been the case in the UK, and other countries, in recent decades.

Volumetric taxation

Tax on alcohol is based on alcohol content of the beverage. Thus, more tax would be paid on a bottle of spirits (40% ABV) compared with a bottle of wine (10–14% ABV) (Cobiac *et al.*, 2009). The level of taxation would be the same when comparing an expensive malt whisky with a cheaper brand spirit.

Differential or targeted taxation

Specific beverages are targeted and taxes increased: for example, alcopops, ciders, tonic wines. Muller *et al.*'s (2010) study on increased taxation on alcopops, in Germany, found that drinkers switched to consuming spirits and an increased preference for beverages associated with riskier drinking patterns. They conclude that, to be effective, policies designed to prevent alcohol-related problems should focus on the control and regulation of total alcohol consumption, as opposed to single beverages.

Ban on price-based promotions
This option refers to restrictions on alcohol sales as loss leaders as well as 'three for the price of two' promotional offers. This is a common element in policies seeking to eradicate cheap alcohol and is broadly supported by the UK Government.

Minimum unit pricing
This involves the fixing of a minimum price for a unit of alcohol applied to either or both the purchase of alcohol on licensed premises (e.g. a public house or club) or off-licensed premises (e.g. a supermarket or off-licence) (Booth *et al.*, 2008; Meier *et al.*, 2010).

Set floor price
This is a variation on minimum pricing based on the 'basic cost of production plus duty plus VAT'. Set floor pricing was a counter proposal, by the Scottish Parliamentary Labour Party (Alcohol Commission, 2010), in response to minimum unit pricing proposals by the SNP administration (Scottish Government, 2008c).

The Sheffield studies
In a review of pricing policies, Booth *et al.* (2008) conclude that there was limited understanding of the effects of pricing on different purchasing and consumption patterns among subgroups of the population. Investigations into alcohol pricing policy options were commissioned by UK Government to investigate the impact of alternative policies on priority groups, namely underage (i.e. under the age of eighteen), eighteen- to twenty-four-year-old binge drinkers and harmful drinkers (i.e. those consuming in excess of the recommended safe limits). The resultant research publications are widely known as the Sheffield studies having been conducted at the University of Sheffield (Booth *et al.*, 2008; Brennan *et al.*, 2008; Meier *et al.*, 2010).

Based on the literature confirming links between price, consumption and problems (Babor *et al.*, 2003; Wagenaar *et al.*, 2009), Meier *et al.* (2010) sought — in an economic modelling study — to consider how different price control options compared, in relation to reducing harm at a population level and to measure the impact of differing policy options on different population subgroups. These studies were innovative in that they considered the heterogeneity of the population, as an important dimension of effect, and they created the opportunity for policies to be more sophisticated and targeted (Room and Livingston, 2010). Subgroups were examined by age, gender and three consumption levels as well as by considering beverage type, price and place of purchase. They showed that, whilst alcohol policies may appear similar at a population level, the subgroups are affected differently by alternative policies.

Table 3.2: Percentage reduction in alcohol consumption for selected policy options: by drinker subgroup and gender.

Policy intervention	Total population	Hazardous drinkers	Hazardous under 25	Harmful drinkers	Males	Females
General price increase:10%	4.4	4.7	6.0	4.5	4.4	4.4
Minimum price 50p	6.9	5.9	3.0	10.3	5.6	9.3
Minimum price 40p	2.6	1.8	0.7	4.5	2.2	3.5
Total ban off-trade discounting	2.8	3.1	0.9	3.2	2.1	4.1
Minimum price 30p/80p off-/on-trade	2.1	1.9	7.2	2.5	2.5	1.4
Low-price on-trade: 25% increase	0.6	0.2	6.1	1.1	0.4	0.9

Source: Meier et al., 2010

Table 3.2 shows the alcohol pricing policy options with the greatest impact. Policy options resulting in a 4%, or greater, reduction in consumption are shaded, indicating the impact on particular target groups. A general price increase of 10% would reduce consumption in the total population between 4.4% and 6.0%, including all target groups and is consistent with the international review on the subject (Wagenaar et al., 2009), discussed above. The total population is clearly influenced by forty and fifty pence minimum unit pricing and the general 10% price increase. However, the impact on the total population is less than the impact on the target groups, with the exception of hazardous drinkers under twenty-five year old. The 'total population' is not a proxy for the 'ordinary' or 'moderate drinker' as it includes those drinking at hazardous and harmful levels. Therefore, the impact of price changes on moderate drinkers would be less than the 'total population'.

Harmful drinkers, including those dependent on alcohol, would be most affected by minimum unit pricing at forty or fifty pence per unit and general 10% price increase. An estimate by Meier *et al.* (2010) of a 4.5% reduction in consumption among harmful drinkers is greater than the 2.8% predicted by Wagenaar *et al.* (2009) regarding 'heavy alcohol consumers'. A total ban on off-trade discounting would have the greatest impact on women, whose consumption would reduce by 4.1%, indicating that women buy alcohol commonly from off-sales, including supermarkets. Hazardous drinkers, under the age of twenty-five, would be most affected by a 'minimum price thirty pence (off-trade) and eighty pence (on-trade)' or 'low price on-trade products price increase of 25%'. This reflects the extent to which younger people drink in pubs and other licensed premises.

That specific pricing policies would affect different groups, in a variety of ways, indicates both the flexibility and sensitivity of such approaches on a range of population subgroups and their distinctive alcohol purchasing and consumption patterns. Policy options are not mutually exclusive; therefore, options could be implemented in combination to maximise the impact on different priority target groups.

Government action

As a result of increased alcohol consumption, and the resultant health and social costs, the price and availability of alcohol have become a matter of public concern, unlike other periods in history when lower consumption and fewer problems were broadly tolerated. In the UK the chief medical officers for all four countries support minimum pricing for alcohol. Similarly, ministers in all UK countries support some form of alcohol price control. The UK Government coalition agreement suggests a ban on below-cost sales of alcohol and a commitment to review both taxation and pricing. In contrast, the Scottish Government has taken a strong line on minimum unit pricing with the clear intention to implement such a policy as a contribution to reducing alcohol-related harm in Scotland. Two potential proposals to tackle alcohol-related problems by controlling price are outlined below.

ALCOHOL PRICE FIXING: examples of proposals to use price as a means to control alcohol consumption in the UK

No. 1: 1979

In 1979 the Central Policy Review Staff (Bruun, 1982) reported confidentially to the UK Labour government on alcohol policies in the UK. Among their recommendations to government were that the 'government should announce a positive commitment on countering the rise in consumption levels and on the reduction of alcohol-related disabilities' and 'the trend towards making drink cheaper as a result of the lag of revenue duties should be arrested: as a minimum duty levels should be kept in line with the RPI (retail price index) (Bruun, 1982, p. viii).

Further, 'given the various ways the government is involved in alcohol policies, not to take a view on desirable per capita consumption is to accept as tolerable whatever levels of disability may ensue' (Bruun, 1982, p. 90). The recommendations were not taken up by government in the following decades.

No. 2: 2010

The policy option of minimum unit pricing (Scottish Government, 2008c) was drawn from the policy modelling studies conducted at the University of Sheffield, which were commissioned by UK Government.

In 2010 the devolved Scottish Government (a minority Scottish Nationalist Party administration) sought to introduce minimum unit pricing as part of a range of measures to influence Scotland's relationship with alcohol and reduce alcohol-related consequences. This element of the Alcohol (Scotland) Bill was defeated, with an acknowledgement by opposition political parties that pricing policy remained a key element in future alcohol policy. The SNP administration, re-elected in May 2011 with a majority, introduced the Alcohol(Minimum Pricing) (Scotland) Bill in November 2011.

In 1979 the Central Policy Review Staff (CPRS) were reflecting concerns about alcohol-related consequences at a time when per capita consumption of alcohol was at its highest since the early years of the twentieth century. During the 1980s many in the policy community, which revolved around the DOH, advocated the use of price and taxation in order to reduce consumption and alcohol-related harm. This did not receive political support (Thom, 1999).

The minimum pricing debate in the first decade of the twenty-first century could scarcely be more different. Current interest in controlling alcohol problems by price is the outcome of a number of years of high levels of consumption, much higher than in 1979, and increased public, media and political concerns about binge drinking, public disorder, health damage and costs. The Sheffield studies were commissioned by UK Government and the policy option formed part of a public consultation (Scottish Government, 2008c) and now inform the Alcohol (Minimum Pricing) (Scotland) Bill (2011). Whilst the commitment to implement minimum unit pricing in Scotland is clear and may exceed that of other countries in the UK, this may reflect the higher burden of alcohol-related harm in Scotland compared to the rest of the UK.

Conclusions

The link between price, consumption and related-health consequences is well established in the international research literature. Consequently, an increase in the price of alcohol will generally result in reduced consumption and in turn related harm. A reduction in the cost of alcohol will result in increased consumption and harm. The relative price of alcohol may be influenced by a variety of economic factors.

In the UK the main concerns about drinking relate to underage drinkers, eighteen- to twenty-four-year-old binge drinkers and older heavy drinkers. The consequent concerns relate to offending behaviour following binge drinking among the younger groups, the health harms associated with hazardous and harmful drinkers and the resulting societal costs. The economic modelling underpinning the Sheffield studies demonstrates the potential to design alcohol price controls, which take account of the heterogeneity of the population on the basis of age, gender, levels of drinking and pricing at on- and off-licensed outlets. Policy interventions may be targeted at specific subgroups, where the impact is greater than in the total population and among moderate drinkers. The nature of the policy options chosen will depend on the level of concern raised regarding specific subgroups and harm within the population. It is likely that a national alcohol pricing policy may consist of a variety of pricing elements, which are not mutually exclusive. An important feature of 'minimum unit pricing' is that beverage price is protected whereas increased taxation may be subject to absorption, by retailers, thereby sustaining lower prices.

Public health concerns have not been the major factor guiding UK tax or pricing policy on alcohol. If price regulation for public health purposes was accepted by governments, they would still have to balance this with the desire to maintain revenue raising and pressure from commercial vested interests. However, public health measures to reduce consumption and governments' desire to raise income are not mutually exclusive and may make price control for public health purposes more palatable to commercial interests.

A view held strongly in the public health field is that a failure to tackle alcohol pricing in the UK will simply continue the levels of alcohol-related damage within the population and fail to resolve the costs to public services dealing with health and social consequences. The proposed policy impacts of price regulation on alcohol are modest, in comparison to the large increases in per capita consumption and harm since the 1970s. The pricing of alcohol as a means of reducing harm appears to be firmly on political agendas across the UK in the early years of the twenty-first century, particularly in Scotland: 'We know of no other preventive intervention to reduce drinking that has the number of studies and consistency of effects seen in the literature on alcohol taxes and prices' (Wagenaar *et al.*, 2009).

In the next chapter prevention of alcohol-related consequences in Scottish drinking culture will be further examined by considering the physical availability and the drinking environment, as influenced by liquor licensing regulations.

CHAPTER 4

Controlling the Drinking Environment

This chapter will consider the regulation of the drinking environment. In particular, there will be a focus on licensing law as it pertains to licensed premises, off-sales and their potential role in reducing alcohol-related harm. Responses to drunkenness and antisocial behaviour in and around licensed premises and in public places will be discussed within the context of outlet density and policing the night-time economy.

The drinking environment is defined broadly. Traditionally, the drinking environment is considered to be the premises where alcohol is bought and consumed: for example, pub, club. As the largest proportion of alcohol purchased and consumed in Scotland is purchased from off-sales so both the local neighbourhood and family home may also be considered to be drinking environments. It should be borne in mind that a drunken incident for an individual, irrespective of consequences, may involve drinking in licensed premises as well as in other settings. This raises the question as to what extent hazardous or harmful drinking can be controlled by licensing regulations.

Liquor licensing

> A consistent theme in the literature is that prevention regulations directed toward commercial sellers and backed up with enforcement are more effective than prevention programs relying solely on education or persuasion directed toward individual drinkers (Babor *et al.*, 2003, p. 133).

In 2007 there were more than 17,000 liquor licences in force in Scotland, a 3% decrease since 1998. The largest decrease, around 15%, was in hotel licences. In the same period there was a 60% increase in 'refreshment licences' (cafes) and 1% increase in restaurant licences. The largest proportion of licences was for off-sales (37%) and public houses (30%). Over the period 1998–2007 off-sales licences changed little: 6,337 in 1998 and 6,232 in 2007 (Scottish Government, 2011a). However, in the early part of this century some licensed premises have increased in size into establishments catering for many more drinkers than the average local pub. Since 2007 major off-sales chain stores have ceased to trade, losing out to supermarkets' discounting prowess:

> The past decade has seen high-street, off-licence chains all but disappear, with the likes of Threshers, Victoria Wine, Bottoms Up and Unwins all going the way of Woolworths … Supermarkets now dominate wine sales: almost three-quarters of all wine sold in the UK goes through the tills of Tesco, Sainsbury's and co, their economies of scale driving down prices and destroying much of the opposition. (Williams, 2011, p. 65)

Liquor licensing in Scotland in the late twentieth century

In Scotland during the 1960s and 1970s licensing hours for public houses were relatively restrictive: pubs closed in the afternoon, at ten o'clock in the evening and were closed on Sundays. A review of licensing law (Clayson, 1972) proposed liberalisation of opening hours, which sought to make drinking environments more family friendly and thereby minimise binge-style drinking and aggression amongst some male patrons of pubs. The overall aim was to civilise drinking habits and eradicate the 'drunken Scot' image of accelerated drinking towards closing time, described as the 'ten o'clock swill' or 'beat-the-clock drinking'.

The Licensing (Scotland) Act 1976 was a landmark piece of legislation both for Scotland and the UK, which began a significant period of deregulation of licensing law across the UK. Legislative changes involved an extra hour's drinking time in pubs, at the end of the day and eligibility to apply for pub opening on Sundays and 'extended hours', covering afternoon and late evening. The result of the uptake of 'extended hours' effectively introduced all-day opening and late-evening opening. Research conducted into consumption patterns, following the licensing changes in Scotland, were neutral in their findings (Duffy, 1992). The absence of any apparent harm associated with liberalised licensing laws in Scotland then formed part of the argument to deregulate licensing in England and Wales in the late 1980s. It is also important to note that the idea of deregulation and individual responsibility for alcohol consumption, and many other matters, were part of the zeitgeist of the 1980s and what has been described as the 'Thatcher era'. Attitudes towards alcohol in Scotland reflected enthusiasm for the licensing changes among the more frequent and heavier drinkers. Negative attitudes were expressed by older people, who would consume less, and by individuals upset by late-night noise, who lived near to late opening licensed premises (OPCS, 1985).

Liquor licensing in Scotland in the early twenty-first century

The Nicholson Committee reviewed Scottish liquor licensing laws and in turn informed the Licensing (Scotland) Act 2005 with a remit to review:

> all aspects of liquor licensing law and practice in Scotland, with particular reference to the implications for health and public order; to recommend changes in the public interest; and to report accordingly. (Nicholson Report, 2003, p. 1)

The 'licensing principles' proposed by the Nicholson Report (2003) became cornerstones of the subsequent legislation: prevention of crime or disorder and public nuisance; promotion of public safety and public health; and protection of children from harm. They reflect the work set out by the *Plan for Action on Alcohol Abuse* (Scottish Executive, 2002), as noted in the guidance to the Act (Scottish Executive, 2007, p. 1). The review was described as a balancing exercise, which took account of many serious causes for concern but which also recognised other considerations that pointed to the desirability of retaining the relatively relaxed licensing arrangements in Scotland (Nicholson Report, 2003).

The Nicholson Report (2003) noted significant changes since the implementation of the Licensing (Scotland) Act 1976. Firstly, the emergence of the 'super-pub', which accommodates considerably more drinkers despite the fact that, at the time of writing, the number of public house licences had remained fairly constant for a considerable period. Secondly, a large increase in the number of off-sale licences over the previous three decades. Thirdly, the widespread granting of 'regular extensions' to permitted hours, which had effectively made the idea of permitted hours redundant, resulting in large numbers of licensed premises being open until very late. It was recommended that 'permitted opening hours' should be abolished, and that there should be no statutorily prohibited hours. Instead, applicants for a liquor licence must specify the hours when they wish the premises to be open. This formed part of the legislation and the guidance (Scottish Executive, 2007), which indicated that up to fourteen hours per day is 'reasonable'. When dealing with a licensee's proposal, the local licensing board were to take account of the licensing principles, consider outlet density and actively include community interests. Scottish licensing legislation is unique in the UK in that there is an overt public health dimension which must be considered by local licensing boards, for which Alcohol Focus Scotland (AFS, 2009) provides supportive guidance.

Off-sales in the community

An off-sales licence is granted in respect of premises alcoholic beverage sold for consumption only off the premises. The *Report of the Working Group on Off-Sales in the Community* (Scottish Executive, 2004) built on the foundations set out by the Nicholson Report (2003). The scope of the review sought better engagement and consultation at community level on the granting of licences and responses which would prevent off-licences being a focus of antisocial behaviour. The review was primarily driven by an 'antisocial behaviour' agenda, whereby there is little reference to the health dimensions of alcohol use. The off-sales referred to are 'corner shop' establishments where the connection between purchase, consumption and conduct may be clear. There was no discussion on large supermarkets as off-sales, despite their significant contribution to the sale of alcohol. The working group investigated why dedicated off-sales and licensed grocers were most frequently used by young people to obtain alcohol and concluded that it was less likely that family grocers would have formal training in place to prevent illegal sales and may be more vulnerable to pressure, including threats of violence. Additionally, it was noted that racial harassment formed part of the pressure to sell alcohol illegally and was targeted at predominantly Asian family businesses. The working group recommended that chief constables give consideration to the priority of their forces in responding to antisocial behaviour around off-sales premises.

Evidence on safer licensed premises

Licensed premises (pubs, clubs) are a focus for alcohol-related offending, including violence, despite the overall decrease in the purchase of alcohol from these settings. Pubs and clubs where alcohol-related aggression and violence occur are often crowded, have frustrated customers because of the slow service, are poorly ventilated and have a lax approach to age limits. It is suggested that creating a safer licensed environment is essentially a regulatory matter where formal enforcement of regulations is required but this is not in itself sufficient (Stockwell and Gruenewald, 2004). Thus:

> effective regulation will ensure that the physical environment is attractive and sends a message to patrons about appropriate behaviour; that it does not irritate or frustrate people by being crowded, excessively noisy, hot or smoky. (Homel *et al.*, 2004, p. 235)

Also, server staff should not tolerate drunkenness or promote intoxication or violent confrontation. Paradoxically, some of the features of 'risky' licensed premises make them attractive to some drinkers. In a study conducted in Edinburgh Black *et al.* (2011) note anecdotally the benefits of licensed premises for harmful and dependent drinkers in that the environment provides control over behaviour, by staff and fellow drinkers, as well as mental health benefits resulting from social contact.

The key elements in a tripartite relationship, involving self-regulation (of the licensed premises), formal enforcement (by police and licensing authorities) and the engagement of local community groups (in consultation and decision-making) were proposed as a means of reducing harm and developing a culture of compliance (Homel *et al.*,

2004). These proposals are broadly consistent with licensing practice in Scotland.

Age restrictions

Age restrictions on the sale of alcohol to young people are intended to limit access in order to prevent alcohol problems including health and antisocial behaviour. In many countries the legal age for purchasing alcohol and consumption on licensed premises is eighteen years of age. In Scotland beer, wine or cider may be consumed on licensed premises by sixteen year olds, with a meal. While it is against the law for someone aged eighteen or over to purchase alcohol for someone under the age of eighteen, it is not illegal for that young person to consume it. It is against the law in the UK to give alcohol to a child under five years of age.

There is a consistent body of research on the impact of public drinking-age laws and alcohol-related consequences. Wagenaar (1993) notes that amendments to the legal drinking age result in changes in a range of problems associated with intoxication (e.g. road traffic fatalities, serious assault, crime and drunkenness) for the age groups affected. Generally, a higher legal drinking age results in relatively lower alcohol-related consequences. Legal-age reduction from twenty-one to eighteen in Western Australia resulted in a substantial increase in rates for serious assaults, when compared with Queensland where the restriction remained in place. Legal-age reductions in New Zealand, from nineteen to eighteen, in 1999, are currently a topic for public and media debate in the light of concerns regarding increased alcohol-related offending, driving accidents and fatalities.

In Scotland, a pilot project and evaluation involved increasing the purchase age from off-sales, for a limited period of time in towns in central Scotland, from eighteen to twenty-one between 5pm and 10pm on Fridays and Saturdays. It was concluded that there had been substantial reductions in antisocial behaviour for the limited duration of the study (Scottish Government, 2008c). This project, in addition to the international research literature on the legal drinking age, resulted in the Scottish Government (2008c) proposing such a change in a consultation document on Scotland's relationship with alcohol. The proposal was defeated as part of the Alcohol (Scotland) Bill in

2010, but it appears that draft guidance on the Alcohol etc (Scotland) Act 2010 indicates that local authority licensing boards could impose an over-twenty-one rule on all off-sales. Public opinion was strongly divided: on the one hand support, whilst on the other strong opposition in the context of the right of sixteen year olds to consent to sex, marry or join the armed services. Perhaps strongest opposition to the notion of increasing the age for alcohol purchase came from the SNP youth wing, who claimed that alcohol problems were not restricted to young people, and the Scottish Youth Parliament which viewed such a development as 'misguided and discriminatory' (Braiden, 2011). Furthermore, those old enough to buy alcohol from off-sales may be more inclined to purchase alcohol for 18–21 year olds. The outcome on this matter has yet to be concluded. Public opinion on age restriction is usually divided; consequently, age limits are difficult to change (Stockwell and Gruenewald, 2004). Irrespective of the age chosen for the purchase of alcohol consistent concern is often expressed about 'underage' drinking. However, the evidence suggests that rigorous enforcement of licensing law and age restrictions has a beneficial effect on underage drinking and associated consequences in that age group. Consequently, there is commonly broad support for the enforcement of current underage drinking laws. The Nicholson Report (2003) and the Licensing (Scotland) Act 2005 confirmed long-standing age restrictions.

Permitted opening hours

Afternoon closure of licensed premises largely disappeared during the 1980s following licensing changes and a broader 'liberalisation'. Evidence on the impact of liquor licensing tended to focus on extended opening hours. In general, increased trading hours are associated with a higher incidence of alcohol-related harm and vice versa (Raistrick *et al.*, 1999).

The main interest currently on permitted opening hours focuses on the potential to control the negative consequences of the night-time economy, drunkenness, assaults, drink driving and hospital admissions. There are few studies on the outcomes of restricting opening hours. In New South Wales (NSW), Australia the judiciary restricted pub closing times to 3am in the city of Newcastle. This resulted in a

37% reduction in assaults when this city was compared with Hamilton, NSW, where no restriction had been imposed (Kypri *et al.*, 2010).

Overall opening hours tend to influence the time and place of drunkenness and associated problems. Very late opening is associated with relatively higher levels of violence and road traffic accidents. Alcohol-related consequences may be reduced by shorter opening hours and even closure of outlets on certain days (Babor *et al.*, 2003). Such findings are clearly in contradiction to the ethos of licensing in Scotland.

Local mix: Outlet density

In a study conducted in British Columbia, Canada, alcohol sales were investigated in relation to increased outlet density and the proportion of liquor stores in private rather than public ownership between 2003 and 2008. They found that a greater number of private outlets per 10,000 of the population were associated with higher per capita consumption: the opposite was the case for government liquor stores. During the study period the policy of privatisation or deregulation of outlets resulted in an increase in private alcohol outlets of around 100%. Furthermore, the percentage of liquor stores in private ownership was associated with higher per capita consumption when density of outlets was controlled (Stockwell *et al.*, 2009).

An Australian study, carried out between 1996 and 2005 in Melbourne, found a clear association between outlet density and domestic violence. Associations were noted for density of pubs (and other on-premise licences) domestic violence and assaults. However, the greatest association was for 'packaged liquor licences', that is off-sales. Livingston (2011) suggests that licensing policy needs to pay more attention to off-licence outlets, including supermarkets. As outlet density does not cause domestic violence, or any other alcohol-related offence, Leonard (2011) acknowledges the relationship between outlet density and domestic violence, and proposes that aspects of the community and social make-up provide explanatory elements in the association between outlet density and domestic violence connection. For example, 'organised' neighbourhoods, whether reflecting social class or level of community activism, may be more effective at reducing or preventing an increase in alcohol outlets. Similarly, a stable neighbourhood or community may withstand an increase in outlets without a subsequent increase in assaults or domestic violence. Additionally, 'transitory' neighbourhoods may suffer greater impact from increased outlet density, particularly off-sales outlets, and in turn increased prevalence of domestic violence. A younger, less-conforming neighbourhood population might in turn attract greater police attention, leading to increased reports of family violence, independent of the impact of outlet density on consumption or domestic violence. Assuming that they have the means to do so, those who are unhappy at such developments in the neighbourhood may move away:

> There is no doubt that the physical structure and the social environment of a geographic area influence individual and family behaviours, and the individuals and families have the ability to change these features, or move. (Leonard, 2011, p. 927)

However, disadvantaged communities are commonly less able to influence policies to their benefit on a wide range of issues.

THE RIGHT LOCAL MIX?

No. 1

Small coastal town with lots of pubs and clubs and close to urban centres. There is a low level of unemployment. The community is heavily dependent on income from tourists, who spend in gift shops, restaurants and bars. There has been a significant increase in the number of cafes applying successfully for refreshment licences, to sell alcohol with food during the day and early evening. The town's attractions are heavily promoted by tourist organisations and local businesses.

No town centre off-sales exist following the closure of a major chain. Two supermarkets are the main source of off-sales alcohol, other than pubs, which are expensive. Town centre disturbance, including violence, when pubs and clubs close around 2am, mainly involves visitors. There are regular high-profile, drunk-driving-related accidents after clubs close as visitors drive home; some of the accidents have resulted in fatalities. There are community groups, which oppose the late opening hours of clubs. Police and the local hospital accident and emergency unit have a brisk trade in dealing with drunkenness and alcohol-related accidents during the summer months and weekends all year round.

No. 2

Post-industrial town with high levels of unemployment and deprivation. There are several pubs in the main street, which sell little food; two of these closed in last two years. Alcohol is bought cheaply from supermarkets and town centre convenience stores.

There is a high level of public drinking, around the town centre, where there is a drinking ban in operation, as well as alcohol-related disturbances at pub closing time. The police are engaged in a range of alcohol-related antisocial behaviour and offending, e.g. domestic disturbances, violence (both domestic and in public). The police and the local hospital accident and emergency unit have a brisk trade in dealing with drunkenness and alcohol-related accidents throughout the week, with a slight increase on weekends.

Considerations

Both towns described in the boxed text reflect recent changes in relation to the closure of small pubs and off-sales, with a move towards drinking out-with licensed premises (at home or in public), and supermarkets increasingly the source of purchase of cheap alcohol. The towns contrast with high unemployment, following industrial closures in one, and low unemployment in the other where tourism and the night-time economy are sources of employment.

Whilst the research literature connects outlet density to health and social problems, the relationship between them is not causal. Scottish licensing guidance (Scottish Government, 2007) notes the importance of outlet density but does not provide an arithmetical solution to the number of outlets in a community. Instead, it devolves this duty to the local licensing board in applying the licensing principles underpinning the legislation. This makes sense given the contrasting features of the towns.

The increased democratisation of the licensing process is important, in that community-based organisations can be more involved in the licensing process, both at the planning and complaint stages. However, the strength of local organisations will be important in making local needs apparent. There is room for conflict on the basis of differing local interests. A group of licensed traders may have different views on licensing matters in comparison to a community council. Licensed traders may have different views from large supermarket chains.

In a country which has deregulated liquor licensing over the last three decades, simply closing outlets may be an unpalatable solution for some, although there is evidence that some have closed owing to economic circumstances.

Both towns generate significant alcohol-related consequences, which require the involvement of police and health services. However, the enforcement of licensing laws, in terms of underage drinking, has a track record of effectiveness. An ecological or whole community perspective is required taking account of the number and density of outlets and their opening hours, as well as community participation and a public health agenda.

Public drinking and public drunkenness
Antisocial behaviour and drunkenness

Restrictions on drinking in public places are designed to reduce the potential for drunkenness and antisocial behaviour, further increasing the public perception that the streets are safe. Many towns and cities across the UK have adopted bans on drinking in public and in Scotland the power to create a local by-law forbidding drinking in designated place has been in force since 1993.

As an example South Ayrshire Council, like many other local councils, introduced a by-law which states: 'any person who consumes alcoholic liquor in a designated place or is found to be in possession of an open container in a designated place shall be guilty of an offence'. The offence is essentially possession and/or consumption, but not drunkenness. Between 1998/9 (9,246 offences) and 2007/8 (26,184 offences) the number of offences under this type of by-law almost tripled. The rise in offences is explained by uptake of such a by-law rather than an increase in offending. Unless other offences were involved these infringements would be dealt with by a fixed penalty notice (FPN).

The introduction of FPNs was designed to enable police to deal with antisocial behaviours more effectively, particularly in the night-time economy, and is consistent with the recommendation to prioritise police attention to nuisance behaviours, particularly around licensed premises (Scottish Executive, 2004). FPN is viewed as providing police with a course of action proportionate to the offence, whilst maintaining police presence on the street:

A large proportion of FPN issued in Scotland — around
62,000 of a total of 65,000 — were used (2007–9) for three
main offences all mainly related to alcohol-related nuisance: 'breach of the peace', 'drinking alcohol in public'
and 'urinating and defecating in public'. (Scottish Government, 2009)

In a survey of police officers 80% considered that most of the people
given FPNs were under the influence of alcohol, commonly around
licensed premises, town and city centres, including public transport
settings. Police officers interviewed were divided on whether FPNs
would result in a long-term reduction in antisocial behaviour (Scottish Government, 2009).

In addition to dealing with alcohol-fuelled antisocial behaviour,
police services have also to deal with those who are drunk and incapable, that is, unable to look after themselves. Under the Criminal Justice
(Scotland) Act 1980, designated places for sobering up are defined as
'a place suitable for the care of drunken persons', where individuals
are taken by police. Service users range from: those who are drunk on
a single occasion and never make contact with a sobering-up service
again; so-called binge drinkers who present on several occasions; and
'chronic recidivists' who are likely to be alcohol dependent and will
present on numerous occasions. The practices involved in sobering-
up services vary greatly across Scotland. In Aberdeen and Inverness
such designated places have a base and operate seven days a week. By
contrast, other areas of Scotland offer a response to local needs, which
may involve triage, first aid, custody nurses, cell monitoring, ambu-
lance and police protocols, accident and emergency services (Griesbach et al., 2009). In the absence of formal sobering-up services the
burden falls to police and NHS accident and emergency staff.

Despite public and policy concerns about binge drinking, drunkenness offences in Scotland have declined from 8,358 in 1998/9 to
6,702 in 2007/8 a reduction of approximately 20%. It is possible that
this trend may be due to altered police practices brought about by
the practicalities of policing large numbers of intoxicated people for
minor infringements. Alcohol is involved in a wide range of offences
where the alcohol element is not recorded in published statistics.

However, it is broadly recognised that alcohol is involved in more than 50% of assaults and breaches of the peace. While most alcohol-related offending may be described as 'nuisance' there is a strong association with serious offences, including serious assault and homicide.

Conclusions

The drinking environment is broadly defined to include licensed premises and drinking in public places, given that consumption is not always confined to one setting. Licensing regulations create enforcement mechanisms available to influence the conduct of the licensed seller: individual independent publican, alcohol trade owned premises, off-licences and supermarkets. In Scotland there is a clear public health objective underpinning liquor licensing. Within licensed premises alcohol-related harm, in particular aggression and violence, may be achieved by reducing overcrowding, effective staff training and responsible service. Some of features of less effective establishments are attractive to some drinkers.

Enforcement of the legal drinking age by licences and police reduces harm. However, there appears to be little support for increasing the legal age of purchase for alcohol. The relatively relaxed licensing arrangements in Scotland contradict the research evidence, which suggests that alcohol-related problems may be reduced by increased age restrictions, limits on permitted hours and closure of outlets on certain days. This places an onus on local licensing boards to apply the licensing principles outlined in the legislation, in order to minimise harm. A tripartite arrangement, involving regulation of licensed premises, formal enforcement by licensing authorities and police, and engagement of community groups, is proposed as an optimum form of collaboration, designed to reduce harm. This is consistent with the ethos of current Scotland licensing regulations.

As a means of responding to drunkenness and antisocial behaviour, restrictions in the form of drinking bans in designated places have been introduced, though the impact of these is unclear. Furthermore, FPNs have been introduced in order to ease the task of policing the night-time economy with little expectation of prevention of further misdemeanours. At this stage the question remains open as to whether current licensing and policing practices will reduce harm.

The following chapters look at change from an individual perspective. However, the practices involved in assisting change exist within a policy context.

CHAPTER 5

Change and Recovery: Whatever It Takes

Disputes regarding the dogma of abstinence or the claim that it is possible to revert to controlled drinking illustrate a deep-seated lack of belief in the individual's chances of changing without treatment. However, when people do change from substance misuse, most of them change on their own. (Klingemann, 2004, p. 161)

One view could be that in truth all recovery is 'natural recovery', with treatment conceived at best as simply the skilful nudging and supporting self-determined change. (Edwards, 2000)

Recovery requires change. Change for the better is synonymous with recovery, irrespective of whether treatment has been part of that process. A significant majority of individuals who develop substance-related problems, including alcohol, tobacco and illicit drugs deal with their problem behaviour without formal intervention or treatment.

The trans-theoretical model (TTM) (Di Clemente and Prochaska, 1998) will be outlined. Research will be evaluated: firstly in relation to what influences drinkers and substance users to change; and, secondly, to consider their motivations for sustaining that adjustment in their recovery journey, whether or not abstinence is the goal. The fundamental nature of change will be emphasised. Evidence of personal resources or recovery capital required to maintain recovery will be explored. The emergence of a 'recovery' movement in Scotland will be considered, including the role of mutual self-help.

With regard to relevant terminology, 'self-change', 'unassisted/unaided change', 'self-quitter' 'natural recovery' and 'spontaneous remission' all refer to the process of changing behaviour without formal help or treatment. 'Spontaneous remission' is a medical term which refers to the reduction in severity of or recovery from any condition in the absence of medical intervention. Similarly, in criminological research 'desistance' refers to a reduction in and cessation of offending. These terms are used interchangeably in the research literature.

A model of change

The most prominent model of change is that put forward by Di Clemente and Prochaska (1998) entitled 'stages in the process of change' or TTM, which has become part of a common language in the health and behaviour change fields. The early research, which informed this model, was based on 'self-quitters' and not treatment service attenders. The model implies that there are distinct stages in making changes and that there are certain processes which are evident to a greater or lesser degree in each stages. The stages are:

- precontemplation: the individual is not considering adjusting their drinking habits and will identify the positive aspects of their drinking, though they are often 'coerced' into services or to consider change by employers, family or the criminal justice system;
- contemplation: the drinker is engaged in considering the 'pros and cons' of drinking and change. For some this may be a period of considerable inner conflict and also of considerable duration;
- preparation: commitment and plans for imminent action to change;
- action: active involvement in changing behaviour and engaging the required resources to support this and prevent relapse, possibly involving treatment;
- maintenance: a stage achieved around six months after 'quitting' or changed behaviour, when the new behaviour is established

and is reinforced by other supportive influences. This would still be described as 'early recovery' by Best *et al.* (2010).

The model also outlines change processes which Di Clemente and Prochaska (1998) describe as 'the engines of change' and the same processes are used with or without formal treatment. Crucially, the model cuts across the artificial distinction between 'self-changer' and 'treatment seeker'.

Table 5.1: Change processes

Change processes	Example
Cognitive	
Consciousness raising*	Look for information on alcohol
Self-liberation*	Self-talk on ability to stop
Social liberation	Awareness of options for non-drinking
Self re-evaluation	Disappointment at continued heavy drinking
Environmental re-evaluation	Negative impact of alcohol on the environment
Dramatic relief	Emotional response to health warnings or portrayals of drinking problems
Behavioural	
Counter-conditioning	Engage in alternative activities
Stimulus control	Remove things from environment or avoidance of e.g. favourite pub and heavy drinking friends
Reinforcement management	Plan rewards: reinforcement from others for moderation or abstinence
Helping relationships*	Having someone who listens

* Most commonly used change processes

Few change processes are evident for those in the precontemplation stage because change is not under consideration. Cognitive processes are more evident among those individuals in the contemplation and preparation stages, whilst behavioural processes are more commonly used in the action and maintenance stages. The most commonly used processes (marked with an asterisk in Table 5.1) are 'consciousness-raising', 'self-liberation' and 'helping relationships'. This is an important finding, which confirms that these are very general change processes and not specific to 'addiction' — let alone alcohol problems in particular. Orford suggests that what is most useful about the stages in this model is:

> The way information about processes assists us in explaining why it is that treatment with very different rationales,

> or indeed no treatment at all, may in essence allow the same
> fundamental things to take place. (Orford, 2001, p. 322)

The stages of change model has been criticised on a number of counts. Firstly, the nature of a staged model implies that individuals must complete one stage before moving on or progressing to the next. It appears that the stages overlap to an extent and that it may be less than clear which stage in the process of change an individual happens to be. For some the change process is not linear and stages can be moved through rapidly or even missed out completely. Being at a particular stage predicts nothing about whether an individual will move to the next stage of the change process. Secondly, it has been suggested (Davidson, 1992; Orford, 2001) that the 'processes of change' outlined in the model are more important than the stages. Despite criticisms, the importance of this model of change and its terminology should not be underestimated as it serves an important function in providing a common language across disciplines involved in behaviour change and service delivery. Other models of change are similar to TTM: for example, Vaillant (1983) proposed a model of change consisting of two stages, namely 'recognition' of the problem and doing something about it, followed by 'maintenance' of the new behaviours and access to a support network.

Self-change: Evidence

This section considers recovery in the absence of formal treatment. Self-changers can be difficult to study — not because of lack of numbers but because they cannot be recruited in the same manner as treatment seekers. Additionally, some self-changers may view their former alcohol problems as part of their past from which they have moved on. They are commonly recruited through:

- identification in population studies by fulfilling set criteria (e.g. self-reported dependence and problems measures);
- media recruitment via advertising;
- informal networks: 'snowballing' or word-of-mouth contacts.

It has been suggested that motivation to change occurs when the good things about drinking are outweighed by the bad things and a decision is made to do something about it. This is observable in the action stage of TTM (Di Clemente and Prochaska, 1998).

Lopez-Quintero *et al.* (2011) investigated the probability of remission from nicotine, alcohol, cannabis and cocaine dependence based on an epidemiological survey of 43,093 US adults. A significant proportion stopped: rates for cannabis and cocaine were between 97% and 99%, while those alcohol and tobacco were slightly lower, at around 90%. This indicates the relative difficulty that individuals experience in giving up or cutting down their use of substances which are socially accepted and easily available. Lower remission rates were also associated with mental health issues, indicating that self-change may also be more difficult for some on the basis of their life circumstances.

From a population survey conducted in Clydebank, Saunders and Kershaw (1979) identified 160 individuals who met the criteria of former 'problem drinkers'. When these individuals were followed up they were asked about the reasons for changing their drinking. Family relationships, employment, finances and health were the most commonly reported influences on drinking behaviour and only those with the most severe alcohol problems reported treatment as an influence. These factors are also commonly reported by those in treatment as factors influencing change (Orford and Edwards, 1977). The reasons given for making changes to drinking are consistent with motivational theories (Cox and Klinger, 2004) where 'current concerns' influence decisions to change. Consequently, an absence of 'current concerns' about drinking, would suggest that change was unlikely.

Traditionally, high 'social capital' and a low severity of alcohol-related problems have been assumed to be the key factors in explaining natural recovery. However, Bischof *et al.* (2003) interviewed 178 media-recruited 'self-changers' with the aim of identifying the existence of different characteristics. From those interviewed, three distinct groups were identified:

- high severity of alcohol dependence, low alcohol-related problems and low social support;
- high severity of alcohol dependence, high alcohol-related problems and medium social support;
- high social support, low severity of dependence, low problems and late onset.

The importance of identifying the heterogeneity of self-changers and specific subgroups enables consideration of group differences in relation to both initiation and maintenance of change or recovery. Furthermore, the idea that self-changers are not 'real alcoholics' is contradicted by these findings.

Individuals' reasons for initiating change reflect the notion of the individual moving from the 'contemplation' to the 'action' stage of Di Clemente and Prochaska's (1998) mode. Rumpf *et al.* (2000) compared 176 media-recruited, alcohol-dependent self-changers, with thirty-two derived from a representative general population sample. Those recruited via the media were more likely to be abstinent in the previous twelve months. They were more severely dependent, had greater prior health and social problems. Rumpf *et al.* (2000) suggest sample bias as an important issue in this study. However, it is possible that those most damaged by drinking and dissatisfied with their life changes are more prepared to respond to media recruitment.

In a study of thirty heroin and thirty alcohol self-changers, Klingemann (2004) reports that they generally went through 'a conscious phase of preliminary deliberation', reflecting on life events which were experienced negatively in the previous year. This in turn progressed to more serious motivation for change through additional triggers. They used distancing or avoidance techniques (avoiding the pub, heavy drinking friends and taking a different route home), substitution of alcohol, negative expectancy (the belief that bad things will happen if drinking is resumed) and behaviour management (alternative activities and hobbies) in the early stages of their recovery. Klingemann (2004) concurs with Lopez-Quintero (2011) in concluding that natural recovery seemed to be more difficult for problem drinkers than illicit drug users, as ex-drinkers (or controlled drinkers) continue to be confronted by high-risk situations and easy availability, precisely because of the role and function of alcohol in society, whereas illicit drug use is less culturally integrated.

Staying free of harm

Staying free of alcohol-related harm reflects the maintenance stage in the TTM (Di Clemente and Prochaska, 1998) and refers to the means by which people 'stay stopped' and sustain their harm-free drinking, or abstinence, in the context of a new way of life.

In the USA, Vaillant (1983) studied paths to recovery. They prospectively followed up more than 400 inner-city teenage males over a thirty-year period. More than 25% met criteria for 'alcohol abuse' and just under half achieved at least one year of abstinence. Stable abstinence was associated with greater severity of alcohol 'abuse', or dependence (as Rumpf *et al.*, 2000, note), and finding 'substitute dependencies', new relationships, behaviour modification and engagement with Alcoholics Anonymous (AA), or religious involvement. In terms of pathways to recovery it was identified that treatment and good premorbid adjustment were not predictive of abstinence. Less than one in five was able to return successfully to problem-free drinking and those men also had fewer symptoms of dependence and alcohol-related problems.

Furthermorefollow-up after sixty years found the both cohorts approaching eighty years of age (Vaillant, 2003). More than half were dead — a higher proportion than would expected for this age group — with 32% abstinent and 1% controlled drinking. A further 12% were 'abusing' alcohol, and it was noted that this pattern of consumption could persist for decades, without resulting in remission, death or progression to severe dependence. It was also reported that chronic dependence was rare. Consistent with earlier findings sustained abstinence was best predicted by prior dependence on alcohol and AA attendance.

Humphreys *et al.* (2006) suggest that, just as alcohol dependence can take years to develop, it can often take a long time to be resolved. This may involve several attempts at altering behaviour, which may or may not include treatment. This is posed in contradiction to the much shorter duration of alcohol treatment. Most studies do not support the view that treatment has a lasting impact on the course of alcohol dependence, and naturalistic studies are proposed as a means of evaluating the impact of the myriad influences, in addition to treatment, brought to bear on the individual, including the individual's employment situation, relationships and engagement with self-help/recovery organisations. Additionally, life events, subsequent to a decision to change behaviour, may enhance or negate the individual's situation. However, the implication is that factors that influence the initiation of change may also be highly relevant to the maintenance of changes over time.

Few studies on natural recovery have considered the role of factors relevant to 'staying stopped' (Bischof et al., 2000). By comparing ninety-three natural remitters and forty-two self-help group attenders they found that self-help group attenders informed more people about their former alcohol problems compared to the natural remitters. This resulted in their receiving reinforcement for their efforts to overcome their difficulties and demonstrated higher social engagement to sustain their recovery. They also sought social support more often as a means of coping with craving. However, Bischof et al., (2000) emphasise that there are more similarities than differences among successful recoveries.

Recovery capital refers to the quantity and quality of resources — both internal and external — which can be used to initiate and sustain recovery (Laudet and White, 2008) and is synonymous with 'social capital' (Granfield and Cloud, 1999). It is implied that recovery or social capital at the initiation of change may be different from that at a later stage and that 'capital' can be accumulated over time to support or enhance the new lifestyle, irrespective of whether formal treatment has been accessed. This applies whether abstinence or harm-free drinking is adopted. Earlier literature, not flying under a recovery banner, defined recovery capital in terms such as 'outcome predictors', that is, characteristics, attributes or resources which the individual brings to the change or treatment process. These predict drinking outcome, whether positive of negative; marital satisfaction or cohesion; employment and job status; commitment to change; and supportive non-drinking networks (Orford and Edwards, 1977; Vaillant, 1983). An absence of these predictive characteristics implies low recovery capital and poor recovery or treatment outcome. The same factors are clearly in play when individuals engage positively in the recovery process over time, consistent with TTM 'maintenance stage' (Di Clemente and Prochaska, 1998). Such findings inform a recovery perspective, which recognises that the resolution of addiction is a complex and lengthy process and is likely to involve fundamental changes in personal well-being and social functioning, including the individual's role in society (Best et al., 2010).

Recovery in Scotland

The Scottish ministerial advisory committee on alcohol problems (SMACAP, 2011) states that:

> the recovery movement has a long history within the alcohol field, going back at least 150 years. Its nature has changed significantly over this time, responding to shifts in the way that society has conceived and prioritised alcohol problems. It is an evolving concept which in the past has been appropriated by certain treatments as a shorthand way of describing it. (SMACAP, 2011, p. 17)

Definitions of recovery vary and are dependent on country and culture of origin:

> Recovery is taken to mean the process through which an individual is enabled to move on from their problematic alcohol use, towards a life free of alcohol-related problems and become an active and contributing member of society. (SMACAP, 2011, p. 14)

This is broadly in line with that of Scottish Government (2008a). The Betty Ford Consensus Panel (2007) defines recovery as 'a voluntarily maintained lifestyle of sobriety, personal health and citizenship'. The Ford definition reflects a USA perspective, where there is a stronger attachment to Twelve Step approaches and abstinence as key elements in the recovery journey. In contrast, SMACAP (2011) states that 'recovery is taken to mean a style of service user involvement rather than any particular treatment type' with 'services to be underpinned by a recovery ethos, which supports and builds on individual strengths and assets', thus enabling individuals to move from harmful drinking to a 'life free from alcohol-related problems' (SMACAP, 2011, p. 17). However, none of these definitions necessarily prescribes the methods required to be implemented in order to achieve recovery. In a review of the research evidence supporting recovery, commissioned by the Scottish Government, two dimensions of recovery are proposed: 'remission of the substance-use disorder'; and 'enhancement in global health (physical, emotional, relational, occupational and spiritual)' (Best *et al.*, 2010). There are a number of influences that have contributed to the emergence of a 'recovery' movement in Scotland, some of which are international in nature while others reflect the needs and aspirations of both the UK and Scotland individually as having state social care and criminal justice systems burdened by the impact of substance misuse.

First influence

'Recovery' approaches have emerged in Europe, North America, Australia and New Zealand driven by an appreciation of the limitations of formal treatments and services, in the fields of mental health, physical disability, where empowerment, inclusion, antidiscrimination and self-help are potent themes.

Second influence

The role of the Twelve Step movement, formed in the USA, has had a global impact, where a strong emphasis on abstinence as a cornerstone of recovery is promoted. However, the impact of Twelve Step approaches has influenced a broader range of social and health concerns than simply alcohol or drugs, as a means of focusing on a single issue relevant to the experience of concerned or affected individuals.

Third influence

In the UK the notion of recovery is reinforced by government policy in relation to reducing dependence on the state benefits among those affected by drug and alcohol-related problems (Home Office, 2010). This is further supported by an employability agenda, which seeks to increase social inclusion by making a contribution to society. Around 70% of drug service attenders in Scotland are unemployed, which is considerably higher than for those who are alcohol dependent (ISD, 2011).

Fourth influence

In the UK the recovery movement has been buoyed by criticism of the long-term prescribing of opioid substitutes — methadone in particular — for illicit opioid users and concern at the low abstinence rates achieved. Consequently, there is an implied criticism of 'drug treatment' and of lengthy and inappropriate prescribing of methadone, in particular. Suggestions that drug treatment has 'failed to maximise potential' by 'turning service users into passive recipients' of risk management services (Scottish Government, 2008a) may be valid but the same case is not made for specialist alcohol services.

Fifth influence

Substance use — both licit and illicit — has increased markedly over the last three decades, yet professional groups and statutory bodies have been slow to recognise and respond accordingly. As responses have emerged they reflect the substance user in the light of statutory responses to children and families, criminal, justice and infection control. These emergent dimensions of service response can also represent barriers to accessing services: for example, substance-using parents' fear of removal of children. As a result the person-centred ethos of the recovery movement may have a significant appeal, both as an adjunct to formal interventions and as a means of supporting self-change.

Service implications

It is suggested that a 'recovery' approach will entail significant change in both the pattern of services that are commissioned and in the way that practitioners engage with individuals, as a means of ensuring that longer-term needs are identified at an early stage. Laudet and White (2008) suggest that understanding and promoting recovery will require a paradigm shift, for addiction professionals, from an acute care model to a longer-term approach, and shifting service provision from 'symptoms to wellness'. It is arguable that Laudet and White's comments are more relevant to the health and social care systems of the USA than publicly funded health and social care systems in the UK. Nevertheless, the 'proposed paradigm' shift is reflected in the SMACAP (2011) report on alcohol services in which a recovery perspective is acknowledged and absorbed into recommendations for enhancing the quality of specialist alcohol services.

The recovery approach outlined is positive in that the range of influences brought to bear on the individual in the change or recovery process —health, family and employment, in addition to treatment for some — are acknowledged. Indeed, much of the literature supporting this view has emerged from several decades of follow-up research on natural recovery and treatment outcome among problem drinkers. However, it is also apparent that the emergence of and support for a recovery movement in Scotland, and the UK more widely, is a result of concerns about illicit drug use, where offending, the effect of substitute prescribing, employment and benefit dependence are viewed with greater concern than for harmful or problem drinkers. It may be argued that alcohol problems are being drawn under the umbrella of substance use, as a secondary issue, despite greater numbers of problem drinkers and considerably greater health and social impacts in total.

Mutual self-help

Groups have a powerful effect on individual members by shaping attitudes, beliefs and behaviour and prolonged engagement reinforces and sustains change (Barrie, 1990, 1991). Mutual self-help groups are an important element of recovery by providing support for behaviour change subsequent to, in parallel with and often instead of treatment.

Self-help group members perceive themselves to share a common problem and as a result seek to support each other in the process of resolving the identified problem, whether this concerns alcohol use or another life difficulty. Such groups are led by group members who have achieved their status by their efforts at resolving their own problems, acting as exemplars, whilst supporting the efforts of other members.

Moos (2008) suggests that there are active ingredients in self-help groups, indicating that support, goal direction, group norms, provision of role models, involvement in alternative rewarding activities, with a focus on teaching and developing coping skills and supporting self-efficacy, are some of the active ingredients which are responsible for the positive impact of self-help groups. Self-help groups vary in their aims and methods and operate on the basis of agreed norms for abstinence or moderation, within diverse cultural contexts. The active ingredients outlined by Moos (2008) in relation to self-help groups are broadly similar to 'therapeutic', where a professional worker adopts the role of facilitator (Barrie, 1990, 1991).

Twelve Step approaches

> To its detractors, AA is unscientific, smacks of fundamen-
> talist religion, excludes those who do not espouse its views
> and is not open to other forms of help for alcoholics. To
> its admirers, AA is an organisation made up of winners.
> (Vaillant, 1983)

Twelve Step is the most widely known self-help approach, both
worldwide and in the UK, and it encompasses groups such as Alcoholics Anonymous (AA), Narcotics Anonymous (NA) for drug users,
Alanon (family members of drinkers), Alateen (for children and
young people whose parent(s) have an alcohol problem), Families
Anonymous (family members of problem drug users). Other associated Twelve Step approaches are Minnesota (a residential Twelve
Step intervention) and Twelve Step Facilitation (TSF), an intervention designed to increase access to and engagement in AA. Harris *et
al.* (2003) report more than 3,000 AA meetings per week in the UK,
with 500 taking place in London. Consequently, AA in particular
provides easy access to a support group in urban areas most, if not
every, day of the week.

Whilst sharing the same functions and processes of most self-help
approaches (Moos, 2008), Twelve Step groups, and agencies which
subscribe to this approach, are quite distinct. Firstly, Twelve Step
groups are spiritual in the sense that there is an acceptance of a 'higher
power', which is strongly reflected in the 'Twelve Steps' towards recovery. Secondly, Twelve Step organisations actively promulgate the view
that addiction is a disease that can be arrested only by abstinence.
Whilst this is contrary to the scientific evidence, it stands as a cornerstone of Twelve Step approaches. AA and other groups are, therefore,
based on a belief system. Bufe (1998) suggests that AA is a cult.

Some problem drinkers attend AA without accessing formal treatment. In the absence of professional treatment Humphreys *et al.*
(1995) note two pathways out of drinking problems, in a three-year,
longitudinal follow-up study, and predict the recovery pathway from
initial subject characteristics. Almost half of a sample of 135 subjects became moderate drinkers or stably abstinent and had higher
socio-economic status and social support. Those who subsequently

became abstinent (N=28) were of low socio-economic status, had severe drinking problems and believed their drinking was a very serious problem and relied heavily on AA attendance. Whilst Humphreys *et al.* (1995) note that lower socio-economic status was a feature of AA attenders, as opposed to 'natural recoverers', it is also widely recognised that some high-status groups/professions — doctors, police and lawyers — often hold exclusive AA meetings. In particular, the medical profession have a Twelve Step oriented support network for members with substance problems in the UK.

Project MATCH (matching alcoholism treatment and client heterogeneity) (Babor and Del Boca, 2003) compared TSF, cognitive behavioural therapy (CBT) and motivational enhancement therapy (MET) (see Chapter 7). There was little difference in drinking outcome between the interventions, although TSF appeared best suited to those who were heavily dependent and lacked a supportive non-drinking social network. Recovered problem drinkers, who were therapists, showed no improved results. In comparisons of outpatient treatment and Twelve Step attendance, improvement on 'no treatment' was demonstrated, but no differences emerged between AA-only and out-patient groups at one- and three-year follow-up (Ouimette *et al.*,1998; Humphreys and Moos, 1996). Whilst Twelve Step approaches appear to be effective, superiority over other interventions is not supported. Project MATCH showed poorer outcome for TSF, where high levels of psychopathology were identified. Furthermore, in relation to major depression and substance use it was noted that those attending a Twelve Step self-help group at one- and two-year follow-up were less socially involved and derived progressively less benefit.

In the UK Twelve Step approaches are used as an adjunct or follow-up to treatment. The National Treatment Outcome Research Study (NTORS) on treated problem drug users investigated the use and impact of NA and AA at five-year follow-up (Gossop *et al.*, 2008). Their findings relate only to residential participants (N=142), where there would be a strong emphasis on abstinence. Clients who attended AA/NA after treatment were more likely to be abstinent from alcohol and drug use. It was concluded that Twelve Step groups 'can support and supplement residential treatment as an aftercare resource'

(Gossop *et al.*, 2008, p. 119). Following treatment Twelve Step group attendance resulted in an increase in friendship networks in general as well as non-drinking friendship networks (Humphreys and Noke, 1997; Kaskutas *et al.*, 2002). Post-treatment engagement with AA by problem drinking fathers predicted increased well-being in their children (Andreas and O'Farrell, 2009).

Twelve Step approaches appear to be an effective support to sobriety and relapse prevention subsequent to treatment, or instead of treatment. Whilst this may be in part due to adherence to the belief system promoted by AA it must also be attributable to the support in the non-drinking environment provided by AA meetings and broader social support:

> The therapist must be willing to find out how AA operates and what its beliefs are, and the best way of doing this is to pay a personal visit to an open meeting of AA — a meeting open to all comers — as opposed to closed meetings which are restricted to AA membership. (Edwards, 1982)

Similarly, SMACAP (2011) recommends that specialist services actively develop links with peer-support and self-help organisations.

Individual recovery pathways

The idiosyncratic way individuals react during their recovery pathways reflects the circumstances leading up to their decision to change and the supports available, including treatment for some, to maintain any changes achieved. 'Recovery is essentially the story of each individual's personal journey into abuse or dependence and the path he or she takes finding a way out' (Di Clemente, 2006, p. 81). This is described in the following two case studies.

A TALE OF TWO RECOVERY CAPITALS

Recovery No. 1

John is twenty-eight years old and had a troubled family background resulting in him spending some of his teenage years in care, during which time his drinking and disruptive behaviour were a source of concern. He left school without qualifications, though considered able, and had a poor attendance record. John has little contact with members of his family and these few meetings have often been acrimonious. Subsequently, he did not settle and has spent a significant amount of time homeless or in prison for violent crimes which occurred when drunk and failure to pay fines for other alcohol-related offences. Whilst in prison he has participated in alcohol information sessions; however, on liberation he has frequently re-offended very soon only to return. John seldom makes contact with helping services when released from prison, other than homeless accommodation. He has worked occasionally as a labourer, usually away from his home area and these periods are marked by periods of harm-free drinking and abstinence. John describes these times as feeling like he was 'getting on track'.

His heavy drinking and lifestyle have resulted in John experiencing poor health for a man of his age. He reports symptoms of alcohol dependence and binge drinks for days at a time, or until his money or that of his drinking colleagues runs out. He has early stages of liver damage and may be depressed.

Recovery No. 2

Janice is forty years old. She runs her own small business and is a lone parent having separated from her long-term partner three years ago, who was also her business partner.

She comes from a supportive family and describes her drinking in her teens as 'just like the rest of the girls'. Her parents who live nearby are very involved in the care of her seven-year-old son and are concerned at their daughter's work situation.

Her café/bar business is in difficulty and may have to be wound up. This may be due to the prevailing economic circumstances but it is certainly related to her drinking. She has been quite drunk at work on occasion and is struggling to control the business effectively. She sees drinking as a requirement of her work both in the workplace and also in the socialising and networking and has recently stopped using her car for these events.

She describes her drinking as having increased since soon after the birth of her son and having escalated around the time of her separation, though her then partner was unhappy about her level of drinking. She complains of tiredness and memory loss following drinking at work, in recent months. She has not been in contact with health services for some time.

We cannot assume that both individuals described in the boxed text have a similar motivation to change; however, the following themes are relevant:

- The life experiences and current alcohol-related problems are very different for these individuals. Both gender and social background play a part and the only common theme is that they both appear to drink too much, but resulting in quite different consequences.

- Is change equally feasible for both individuals? This seems unlikely on the basis of the resources that appear to be available to Janice. She has a business and income, a supportive family (and child), who have expressed concern. Broadly, this defines her social/recovery capital. The opposing side to this is that the supports available to her could be diminished or lost by continued drinking and this may be a motivator for change.

- By contrast, John's deprived background and the severity of his current life situation mean that he appears to have very little in the way of social capital, other than a desire to work, allied to periods of sobriety at different points in his life. He appears to have little to lose by comparison. This reflects the tendency for higher levels of social/recovery capital among middle class problem drinkers as a predictor of recovery.

- In both cases attention should be paid to the resources or recovery capital, which they both possess and which need to be mobilised in order to support behaviour change and recovery. An element of recovery that is potentially predictive is that of self-efficacy, that is, the extent to which an individual believes that they are capable of change.

- Janice could be a 'self-changer' enlisting support from those around her to sustain change. Alternatively, she could be a treatment seeker. However, her family and business commitments suggest that help be offered in the context of community-based services or out-patient care and support. Recovery for Janice could involve the retention of her business, family and the support and reinforcement, which all this offers. She may continue to consume alcohol, or may abstain — either way seeking support in that decision and engaging in non-drinking social activities.

- Recovery for John would look quite different given his previous life experiences and supports. John's unstable situation suggests that he is unlikely to be a successful 'self-changer'. Should he decide to opt for more formal help, as a treatment seeker he would commonly be involved in a residential care setting for alcohol problems, frequently described as 'rehabilitation', whereby a wide range of social supports and opportunities might be on offer: for example, individual and group intervention for alcohol dependence plus enhancement of employability and independent living skills. Such services also support Twelve Step meeting (AA) attendance. The opportunity to work would be useful in its own right and as a bolster to abstinence.

- Both may benefit from social support for harm-free drinking or abstinence: whether a Twelve Step organisation would suit as a support for abstinence may be worth exploring. In the longer term 'recovery' needs for each are likely to be very different. Furthermore, in both cases their needs and effective supports are likely to change over time reflecting other developments in their lives: for example, changing family relationships, employment and business opportunities, commitment to harm-free or non-drinking.

- With regard to personal identity it is quite likely that they would have different ideas about whether they would consider or describe themselves as former problem drinkers. The proposed recovery trajectory for John may make it difficult for him to divest himself of the 'recovering alcoholic' label. This would not be the case for Janice given the potential for her to recover without a lengthy recovery trajectory constructed for her by mutual self-help groups and rehabilitation services.

Conclusions

Natural recovery is not the opposite of assisted recovery ('treatment') and the two are intertwined. The common feature is change, a process which underlies all recovery. Consequently, the distinction drawn between self-changers and treatment seekers is false (Di Clemente, 2006). Treatment is time limited and enhances the change process, for some individuals, in the considerably longer recovery journey towards well-being.

Social influences on an individual's decision to change are wide ranging and important. Enduring financial and health problems may be triggers for motivation to change, as can the pressure from family, employers and the criminal justice system; they are also central to the maintenance of change or recovery. The majority of individuals who develop alcohol and other drug problems recover, whether by achieving abstinence or harm-free use, without accessing treatment services. In general, higher socio-economic status and social stability are predictive of the likelihood of recovery from alcohol dependence, which may include a return to moderate drinking (Humphreys, 2006). This may be because of the possession or acquisition of recovery or 'social capital'. By contrast, those from more disadvantaged or deprived backgrounds, and where social instability features, are less likely to fare well. Recovery capital tends to be unevenly distributed between social classes, and harmful drinkers from deprived backgrounds more commonly abstain as part of their recovery. However, in the absence of social capital as an influence on change processes it is then feasible that harmful and dangerous drinking patterns persists with more harms accrued.

Prior high levels of dependence and AA attendance are predictive of abstinence (Vaillant, 2003) and those who achieve controlled alcohol use tend to have been less dependent on alcohol, are younger and more socially stable. Reduction in harm is an important aspect of recovery, irrespective of whether the drinking goal is that of control or abstinence. Pathways to recovery are highly individualistic. In essence, the individual's new harm-free behaviour is regulated by social norms that reinforce moderation and selectively punish the possibility of excess: for example, by maintaining contact with family and friends who provide a 'non-drinking' or moderate drinking environment. The use of support networks, including mutual self-help groups, are an important dimension to maintaining new behaviours, by providing exemplars and support in a harm-free environment.

The debate and literature on 'self-change' are predominantly individually oriented. However, if recovery capital is seen also as a function of the community and society as a whole, then assisting individuals to change may be seen as a function of wider policy, regulatory controls and community involvement. Given the increased difficulties faced by users of legal drugs (alcohol and tobacco) in making changes, policy initiatives to curb consumption by regulation of availability, price and access to brief interventions become crucial elements in supporting change on hazardous and harmful drinking.

It remains to be seen whether change and recovery from

alcohol-related problems will be enhanced by the recently emerged recovery movement. Its importance lies in an ability to take a longer-term view of recovery and encourage the development of innovative means of support and the enhancement of support or social capital both at community and individual levels. This perspective may in turn influence the nature and style of the delivery of treatment for alcohol-related problems. On the one hand influences have been clearly drawn from the 'addiction' change, recovery and treatment research literature, whilst on the other UK government policy on employability and the reduction of dependence on state benefits have become bed-fellows, which drive the recovery agenda. This is further reflected in Scottish Government's (2008a) policy document on recovery, the title of which refers to Scotland's 'drug problem'. The 'recovery' movement in Scotland appears to be driven more by concerns surrounding illicit drug use than by concerns of harmful or hazardous drinking despite the greater damage inflicted by alcohol.

The themes of change and recovery underpin, and are developed further in, Chapter 6, where ABIs for hazardous and harmful drinkers will be addressed, while Chapter 7 will review the role of specialist treatment for dependent harmful drinkers.

Alcohol Brief Interventions

> Much work remains to be done before BI is considered to
> be an integral part of mainstream preventive medicine and
> public health. (Nilsen, 2010, p. 957)

Alcohol brief interventions (ABI) are an element of public health
and preventive responses which reflect the broadening conception of
alcohol-related problems, beyond the narrow focus on dependence
or addiction, and are therefore based on the notion of targeting large
populations of hazardous and harmful drinkers, and intervening
at an early stage. Given the large numbers of drinkers who may be
contacted opportunistically, improvements in both individual and
public health may be achieved.

Screening and brief interventions for alcohol-related problems
should be viewed in the context of stepped care, an initial and opportunistic means of reviewing alcohol consumption and related harm in
the large population of healthcare seekers as opposed to those seeking
treatment for severe alcohol-related problems. In the spirit of stepped
care it is also possible that those with severe alcohol-related problems
may be identified and offered referral to appropriate services. Given
the individual focus of this public health approach behaviour change
is underpinned by the themes explored in Chapter 5.

This chapter will clarify key themes surrounding ABI. Consideration will be given to definitions of brief and 'extended' brief interventions and in turn the target groups for whom ABI can be effective.
The research evidence on effectiveness will be examined, emphasis-
ing the settings in which ABIs may be delivered. The vast majority of

research on brief interventions has taken place in healthcare settings, and there is a significant gap regarding social care and criminal justice. Significant obstacles preventing the delivery of this response to alcohol problems are evident, even in healthcare. Barriers to engagement with problem drinking will be explored.

Screening

The majority of patients in healthcare participate in screening procedures on many health topics (e.g. diet, smoking) that are part of routine practice. The first stage in offering brief interventions involves screening and assessment. Whilst a healthcare professional may offer a brief intervention on the basis of a lengthy health history, or prior knowledge, the aim of opportunistic intervention is to use brief screening questionnaires on large numbers of health service users routinely, and rapidly. The questionnaires outlined below are some of those currently in use in healthcare, based on evidence of their effectiveness in identifying hazardous drinkers, as a precursor to offering ABI and identification and appropriate referral for those harmful drinkers, who evidence alcohol dependence. They are recommended as best practice by the Raistrick et al. (2006), the Scottish Inter-Collegiate Guidelines Network (SIGN, 2003) and the National Institute for Clinical Excellence (NICE, 2010a). The CAGE questionnaire (Mayfield et al., 1974) is widely used; the higher the score the more significant the alcohol problem:

- Have you ever felt you should **C**ut down on your drinking?
- Have people **A**nnoyed you by criticising your drinking?
- Have you ever felt bad or **G**uilty?
- Have you ever had a drink first thing in the morning (**Eye opener**)?

Adaptations of CAGE have been used in prisons (ISD, 2011) and the questionnaire has been further refined for use in antenatal services and preconception consultations: for example, T-ACE (Take number of drinks, Annoyed, Cut down, Eye Opener) (Sokol et al., 1989) or TWEAK (Tolerance, Worried, Eye opener, Amnesia, Kut down) (Russell, 1994). An evaluation of screening questionnaires in antenatal services — T-ACE, TWEAK and AUDIT-C — 'showed promise', while CAGE performed poorly (Burns et al., 2010). In a comparison study

(Hodgson *et al.*, 2003) in UK accident and emergency departments the fast alcohol screening test (FAST), CAGE and the Paddington alcohol test (PAT) (Smith *et al.*, 1996) were all quicker to administer — less than one minute — than the full alcohol use disorders identification test (AUDIT) (WHO, 1996). AUDIT is considered the gold standard and has been subject to alterations to shorten administration time. The lack of research on screening tools validated out-with healthcare makes it more difficult to recommend specific questionnaires for use.

ABIs

A set of principles, informed by cognitive behavioural and motivational methods, have emerged (Raistrick *et al.*, 2006), which suggest that ABI should include the following elements, based on the acronym FRAMES:

- Feedback: on risk and harm from screening, assessment or test;
- Responsibility: emphasis on personal responsibility for alcohol use and change;
- Advice: provision of clear practical advice and self-help material;
- Menu: options for change;
- Empathy: non-judgemental and supportive;
- Self-efficacy: increase individual's belief in their ability to change.

A wide range of ways to deliver ABI have been devised and tested, including brief counselling, written materials, self-help manuals, motivational interviewing (Robertson and Heather,1998; Dunn *et al.*, 2001; Carey *et al.*, 2011) and more recently on-line interactive versions are available (Kaner *et al.*, 2002). In an evaluation of the impact of strategies promoting screening and brief intervention by nursing professionals, three interventions were investigated; written guidelines (control group); outreach training; and training with telephone-based support. The two experimental groups demonstrated higher levels of use in routine practice. Despite this, the control group was more accurate in their application of their intervention and made fewer errors. Overall, the balance of evidence is suggestive of the use of written guidelines by nurses in primary care.

How brief is brief?

Raistrick *et al.* (2006) outline two types of intervention, which are best seen as a continuum of increasing engagement. Whilst the distinctions may appear arbitrary, the crucial feature of these approaches relates principally to the settings in which they can be delivered and what is feasible given organisational constraints, including time. Simple brief interventions consist of giving structured advice taking no more than a few minutes to deliver. This is sometimes described as 'minimal intervention'. Poikolainen (1999) considers the distinction between very brief interventions (5–20 minutes) and 'extended' brief interventions, involving several contacts. No difference between men and women was noted for very brief interventions and only women benefited from extended brief interventions. Extended brief interventions consist of structured therapies or psychosocial interventions which may take up to thirty minutes, possibly involving further interventions. MET, one of the interventions tested in Project MATCH (Babor and Del Boca, 2003) and UKATT (United Kingdom alcohol treatment trial, 2008) for dependent drinkers, was delivered in less than four hours and is sometimes referred to as a brief intervention. The duration of a brief intervention is most likely to be driven by the feasibility of offering the intervention in the context of organisational and workplace demands: for example, a brief intervention may be different in content and duration in an accident and emergency department when compared with a general medical ward or a criminal justice setting.

Evidence for ABIs

In an Australian study of the cost-effectiveness of strategies to reduce alcohol problems brief interventions, as one of a number of approaches, was considered a positive response to the prevention of alcohol-related disease and injury (Cobiac *et al.*, 2009; SIGN, 2003; NICE, 2010a).

ABIs are commonly delivered opportunistically in a variety of healthcare settings. With a large body of research on brief interventions since the early 1980s a significant number of overviews of research have been conducted. Their findings are broadly similar, in that they conclude that brief interventions are beneficial to the health of hazardous or harmful drinkers and to public health. Therefore, ABI should be restricted to those with problems of relatively low severity and this is further confirmed by systematic reviews (Bien *et al.*, 1993; Dunn *et al.*, 2001; Moyer *et al.*, 2002; Slattery *et al.*, 2003; Babor *et al.*, 2006). The Mesa Grande systematic review (Miller *et al.*, 2003) ranks ABI at the highest level, based on a substantial research track record of modest but positive outcomes, and this is reflected by the National Treatment Agency (England and Wales) (NTA) recommendations on responding to alcohol problems in the UK (Raistrick *et al.*, 2006).

The majority of the population in the UK access healthcare via primary care services including general practitioners. 'General practitioners and other primary healthcare staff should opportunistically identify hazardous and harmful drinkers and deliver a brief (ten-minute) intervention', according to the Scottish Inter-Collegiate Guidelines (SIGN, 2003). In a USA study, more than 600 adults over the age of fifty-five were randomly assigned to receiving a booklet on health behaviours (control group) or an intervention, which included personalised feedback, information on alcohol and ageing, a drink diary and telephone advice over a period of up to eight weeks. It was concluded that at the twelve-month follow-up there was no reduction in the proportion of heavy drinkers in the sample; however, there was evidence that there was a reduction in alcohol consumption (Moore *et al.*, 2011).

Central to this approach is that of impact, or effect size. The 'numbers needed to treat' (NNT) is defined as the number of hazardous or harmful drinkers who need to receive an intervention for one drinker to reduce their consumption to within recommended limits. The NNT for ABIs is eight (Moyer *et al.*, 2002), whereas the NNT for smoking is ten, if nicotine replacement therapy is used as part of the intervention. Therefore, ABIs in a primary care setting represent both effectiveness and good use of resources.

In an accident and emergency setting in the USA, Gentilello *et al.* (1999) evaluated brief interventions as a routine component of trauma care. Those screened as 'alcohol positive' were randomly allocated to a brief intervention or control group. At twelve months, the group receiving the brief intervention had reduced their consumption significantly more than the control group. Those with mild to moderate alcohol problems were more likely to have reduced their consumption. Following brief interventions, there was a 47% reduction in injuries requiring emergency or trauma centre admission and a 48% reduction in injuries requiring hospital admission. In a similar study of a brief intervention based on the principles of motivational interviewing (Mello *et al.*, 2005), a brief motivational intervention for alcohol plus a booster session showed a reduction in subsequent trauma at one-year follow-up of non-critically injured patients in a trauma centre, whose alcohol consumption had been hazardous or harmful.

In the UK Crawford *et al.* (2004) investigated the impact of a screening and brief intervention that had been incorporated into practice in an accident and emergency department. The experimental group received a leaflet and a thirty-minute, patient-centred discussion on their alcohol consumption, with a health worker, while the control group received only a leaflet. Significant reductions in consumption were evident at six- and twelve-month follow-up in the experimental group. As with other accident and emergency service studies a reduction in demand was observed. A review of research by D'Onofrio and Degutis (2005) on brief interventions in emergency and trauma services in the USA concludes that screening and brief interventions for alcohol-related problems were effective and that they should be incorporated into routine clinical practice. D'Onofrio and Degutis (2005) further report that clinicians in emergency services considered performing a brief intervention to be both feasible and acceptable in everyday practice, in spite of a need to pay attention to specific challenges such as time constraints, ethical and legal issues.

A substantial proportion of patients in general medical wards may be hazardous or harmful drinkers. Raistrick *et al.* (2006) recommend against the use of brief interventions in the general medical wards on the grounds of inconclusive evidence of effectiveness. However, in general medical wards in Edinburgh Chick *et al.* (1985) compared a one-hour intervention by a nurse with a 'treatment as normal' control condition and both groups showed improvement — as might be expected — in alcohol consumption at a time of ill-health, and the brief intervention also demonstrated greater reductions in alcohol-related harm at follow-up.

Chang *et al.* (2005) provide strong evidence in support of screening and ABIs in antenatal care settings. As no universally agreed safe level of alcohol use has been agreed, they suggest that it is useful to modify women's alcohol consumption early in their pregnancy and in turn reduce foetal risks. Chang *et al.*'s brief intervention studies in the USA demonstrated a greater likelihood of abstinence at follow-up and that women with the highest levels of consumption made the greatest reductions. Furthermore, the effect of ABI was enhanced with the involvement of a partner.

Education

At a private residential university in the USA, 667 students were sanctioned for breaking the establishment alcohol policy and were randomly allocated to four experimental conditions, including brief motivational interviewing (BMI), two computer-driven interventions and a control group. Females, but not males, in the control group reduced consumption having received only the sanction. They found that male students reduced their alcohol consumption irrespective of the brief intervention, but did not maintain the change. Female students reduced their consumption to a greater extent after BMI, in comparison to the computer-driven interventions, which was sustained at one-year follow-up (Carey *et al.*, 2011).

A study conducted in inner London further education colleges (McCambridge and Strang, 2004, 2005) compared a control group of sixteen- to twenty-year-old students, with a focus on influencing their drug use, including cannabis, alcohol and tobacco. The extended brief intervention (one-hour session of motivational interviewing) showed a reduction in levels of alcohol and cannabis use at three months, which almost disappeared after twelve months. There was also a reduction in use in the control group. In a Scottish study of further and higher education students, 65% of which were binge drinkers (mean age twenty-three years), a one-hour cognitive behavioural educational session was offered. Subsequently, binge drinkers' positive attitudes towards binge drinking and their intention to binge drink shifted toward the beliefs held by the non-binge drinkers. Binge drinkers persisted in their belief that binge drinking was more prevalent among peers than did the non-binge drinkers (Marks *et al.*, 2011).

Young peoples' alcohol consumption — as characterised by binge drinking and brief interventions — may therefore be concluded to be an important element in any strategy to reduce consumption and consequences. The evidence indicates that brief interventions have a positive impact on young people's drinking and drug use, though the duration of impact may be time limited, when compared with older hazardous and harmful drinkers, identified opportunistically in health services, where the impact of ABIs is more enduring. Educational establishments appear to be an appropriate setting for ABIs.

Social work and criminal justice services

The impact of alcohol on social care, social work and the criminal justice system is discussed in some detail in Chapter 2. The potential for brief interventions being delivered within social services targeting children and families and community care clients represents a significant opportunity. The same may be said of the criminal justice system, where alcohol consumption is strongly associated with offending. Brief interventions might form part of the already extensive range of services designed as alternatives to custody (probation, community service) as well as part of the through care and preliberation services provided within the prison system. Whilst it is possible that the principles of ABI have been taken from the healthcare evidence and applied in these settings, there appears to have been no research conducted on ABIs, in the UK, to suggest effectiveness or otherwise.

A study conducted in primary care appears highly relevant to social work services. Brief interventions were offered to family members affected by the alcohol or drug use of a close family member, in the Midlands and south-west England. Relatives (N=143) were randomly allocated to either a full or brief intervention, both of which were delivered by healthcare professionals. The 'full' intervention consisted of up to five sessions, using a structured manual focusing on substance use, stress coping and support; in addition, the family member was provided with a self-help version of the intervention manual. The brief intervention consisted of one session, during which the content of the self-help manual was explained and the family member was encouraged to make use of the manual, in their own time. Stress and coping measures at the twelve-week follow-up showed no difference between the two groups. It was concluded that a well-constructed self-help manual delivered by a healthcare professional was likely to be as effective as several face-to-face contacts between health professionals and family members (Copello *et al.*, 2009).

Barriers: The workforce

Despite clear evidence of effectiveness for ABI, efforts to encourage health professionals to incorporate screening and ABI in their professional repertoire have met with limited success. As a result a significant research literature has emerged investigating the obstacles to implementation. Since the 1970s, research has confirmed the reluctance of nurses, doctors and social workers, out-with specialist addiction services, to deal with alcohol problems (Shaw *et al.*, 1978; Kaner *et al.*, 1999; Watson *et al.*, 2011). The key findings suggested that workers lacked:

- role adequacy: worker's perception of having the knowledge and skills to work with problem drinkers;
- role legitimacy: the perception that working with problem drinkers is part of their professional task;
- role support: having someone within the organisation who can provide advice support and guidance.

It was noted that training events designed to fill a gap in professional education could increase the confidence regarding knowledge and skills of health and social workers; however, motivation to engage remained low (Barrie, 1992). In comparing social workers with mental health nurses Lightfoot and Orford (1986) conclude that social workers experienced a greater level of 'situational constraint' and in turn less therapeutic commitment to working with problem drinkers. Organisational constraints consisted of time restrictions, lack of supervision or guidance and low priority for working with drinkers. Attempts to influence situational constraint, by training social works and their managers in Scotland, resulted in greater role support and legitimacy, which was sustained, among those workers whose manager had received training (Duffy *et al.*, 1998). However, these innovative postprofessional-qualification training ventures could never influence the curricula of the various professional

training regimes, which appeared to (and still do) pay little attention to substance-use issues. In a survey of social work students,
89% thought that the social work degree should include training on
substance-use problems, supporting long-standing views of a British Association of Social Workers (BASW) special interest group. In
response, a representative of the Social Work Reform Board suggested
that the topic must be weighed against many other pressing curricu-
lum demands (Professional Social Work, 2011). A major conclusion
in Galvani and Forrester's (2011) review of evidence on social work
and recovery for the Scottish Government was that formal social
work education had failed in preparing social workers for working
with substance-use issues. Similar themes are raised by Watson *et
al.* (2011) with regard to nursing. It would appear that opportunities have been missed, to provide greater attention to substance-use
issues, during a period when both nursing and social work qualifications increased study duration to degree level. Scottish Government
and the Convention of Scottish Local Authorities (COSLA) (2010)
identify the need to set out learning priorities and competencies for
all levels of the workforce on alcohol and drug issues and acknowledge the need for strategic leadership, nationally and locally.

In a multi-centre European study, which included a Scottish
cohort, Gilchrist *et al.* (2011) conclude that health professionals,
nurses, doctors, social workers considered working with substance
users to be of lower status than helping other patient groups. Lower
status still was accorded to working with drug users compared to
drinkers. Substance users were seen to be less appealing, in particular
to staff from primary care, when compared with general psychiatry
or specialist addiction services. Clearly, the workforce in primary care
requires considerable support in order to be convinced that working with substance-use issues — alcohol included — is a worthwhile
and relevant activity. The root of such barriers to using ABI lies in
both the health and social policy arenas, whereby the relevance of ABI
to improving public health has not been underpinned by adequate
resources and procedures. This is reflected in the professional education of those commonly in contact with hazardous and harmful
drinking, medicine, social work and nursing, resulting in a sense of
inadequacy and reluctance. Nilsen (2010) notes the professional bar-

riers to implementation and suggests that further research in this particular area is likely to produce diminishing returns, presumably on the basis that the problems have been clearly delineated and now require a solution.

NHSScotland appears to have addressed the stated barriers and implemented a scheme to integrate ABIs into routine healthcare practice, with a target of delivering 149,999 ABIs in the period 2008–11; the target set was exceeded within the deadline (NHSScotland, 2008; Scottish Government, 2011). At this stage the impact of this approach has yet to be evaluated so it remains to be seen whether ABIs will be integrated into routine practice, beyond the project's duration. This policy intervention is in direct contradiction to Nilsen's (2010) suggestion that a 'tops-down' approach to ABI is not the best way forward. However, it is difficult to see how a programme designed to have an impact on health, nationally, could feasibly be delivered other than by centralised policy directive and appropriate resourcing and funding to match.

Conclusions

ABI represents a wide range of methods bound together by the brevity of professional input. There is evidence of a modest but consistent impact on consumption and consequences in hazardous and harmful drinkers, including binge drinkers, who are identified opportunistically, most commonly in healthcare settings. The potential for tackling alcohol issues at an earlier stage, implying lower levels of dependence and less severe and intractable problems, can make a substantial contribution to individual and public health. ABI is not recommended for those who are significantly dependent on alcohol, but is an effective means of identification and access to appropriate services. The evidence is strongest for ABI using a variety of methods both in healthcare settings, including accident and emergency, primary care and antenatal services, and in further and higher education settings. There is a gap in the research on ABIs in social care and criminal justice.

Barriers to delivery have been identified to implementation of alcohol screening and ABI in primary healthcare, including lack of time and lack of suitable reimbursement. Inadequate professional training may contribute to the reluctance of professionals to engage with brief interventions and alcohol problems more generally. Training and support can increase implementation and should be carefully adapted to meet the needs and attitudes of the workforce. The overall aim is to build the role adequacy and legitimacy among staff in generic/non-alcohol specialist services to deliver ABI. The evaluation of NHSScotland's ABI project will shed light on ways forward. However, given that improvement in public health is a consequence of competent policy and resourcing, the future of ABIs rests with the policymakers and their enthusiasm and ability to overcome the obstacles and make the delivery of a public health benefit a reality.

Some of those identified by alcohol screening may not be suitable for ABI, because of their level of harm and dependence on alcohol. The next chapter will focus on those individuals who may opt for specialist treatment as part of their recovery.

CHAPTER 7

Specialist Treatment/Interventions

> Habit is habit and not to be flung out of the window by any
> man, but coaxed down stairs a step at a time (Mark Twain).

In this chapter specialist treatment for alcohol problems, or dependence, is set in the overall context of change and recovery (see Chapter 5). This implies that treatment alone is not sufficient to resolve dependence on alcohol and associated problems on a sustainable basis. From the wide range of alcohol problems experienced in the population some people — but not all — seek and require specialist help in order to resolve their alcohol-related problems, including dependence. The characteristics of 'treatment seekers' will be identified and considered in relation to treatment outcome and recovery capital. The research that underpins current evidence-based practice will be evaluated by exploring reviews of specialist alcohol treatment studies, client-treatment matching studies and pharmacological interventions. A critique of alcohol treatment research will be developed, based on the similarities in outcome from different treatment interventions, which point to common change processes.

Scottish alcohol needs assessment

Studies by Drummond *et al.* (2005, 2009) sought to quantify the gap between the prevalence of dependence in the population and the availability of specialist alcohol treatment services. The prevalence of alcohol dependence in Scotland was 4.9% in adults over sixteen years of age, affecting 206,000 people. Males had approximately twice the prevalence of alcohol dependence when compared with females (6.7% and 3.3%, respectively). This represents a lower male to female ratio (2:1) in Scotland than in England (3.4:1). The prevalence of male alcohol dependence is quite similar in Scotland and England (6.7% and 5.8%, respectively) but the female prevalence is approximately double in Scotland compared to England (3.3% and 1.7%, respectively). The higher prevalence rate overall for alcohol dependence in Scotland is largely accounted for by the higher prevalence of alcohol dependence in women.

The prevalence of alcohol dependence ranged from 4.3% in Grampian and Tayside to 6.1% in Greater Glasgow. The estimated number of people accessing alcohol treatment per annum in 2006/7 was approximately 17,000 of the 206,000 estimated to be affected, that is, one in twelve per annum, compared with one in eighteen per annum in England. A lower ratio indicates greater access to treatment in Scotland, though in both countries there was significant variation between health board areas (Drummond *et al.*, 2005, 2009). It is recommended in both studies that services should be available to provide a treatment service to 15% of the affected population per annum, which is consistent with North America. This is a modest recommendation and takes account of the fact that a significant proportion of those affected will not access treatment services.

Treatment seekers

Differences between treatment seekers and self-changers are neither dramatic nor consistent (Di Clemente, 2006). Given what is known about change and 'natural recovery' (see Chapter 5) it is important to have an understanding of why anyone would want to seek treatment for an alcohol problem, as opposed to resolving it themselves. Treatment seekers are commonly people who have experienced prolonged problems and have been unsuccessful at self-change and feel the need, or are motivated by others, to seek help out-with their own social network. For severely dependent and chronic drinkers it is clear that greater complications and additional problems (difficulties with relationships, health, employment, offences and control over drinking) can make natural recovery more difficult and contribute to a decision to seek help. Treatment seekers tend to have lower levels of personal and social capital and greater levels of vulnerability (Best *et al.*, 2010).

Those opting for treatment are commonly at different stages in the process of change (see Chapter 5). Some may feel that they are coerced into treatment by family, the criminal justice system or other forces and that seeking treatment was their only option; they may be 'precontemplators' and potentially quite resistant to change and may simply seek relief from stress and discomfort. Some may maintain a view that alcohol is not the main problem in their life or will have come to the conclusion that their drinking is causing problems for themselves and others but may be unsure of what to do about it. Others may be clear about their goals and seek support and skills in order to stay abstinent or drinking without harm. Whilst client characteristics such as social or recovery capital are important predictors of treatment outcome, it is not uncommon to find individuals in specialist alcohol services who have lost a great deal in life, through drinking, and who consequently have few of the resources and opportunities available to them. The absence of these resources predicts poor treatment or recovery outcome and in turn may increase dependence on treatment services.

Opting to seek treatment can be difficult. In a review of studies on unassisted change, stigma and embarrassment formed a major barrier to accessing treatment, as did negative beliefs or experiences of treatment (Sobell *et al.*, 2000). These themes are also reported by those accessing treatment who commonly report the practicalities of family life, child care and service accessibility as barriers.

Specialist treatment

Specialist treatment for severe alcohol problems is predominantly psychosocial in nature, based on talking therapies, plus the appropriate use of pharmacological interventions as an adjunct. Consequently, treatment should be person centred (Scottish Government, 2010b). Despite a wide range of named therapies the primary elements of specialist treatment are assessment, psychological interventions and pharmacological interventions.

Assessment consists of:

- reviewing medical, social and psychological risk and harm (to self and others);
- judging and enhancing the motivation for change: social capital;

- matching need to suitable services.

Psychosocial interventions are used to:

- motivate the individual to engage in a change/treatment process;
- support motivation and enhance self-efficacy;
- provide skills and supports which will enhance the individual's lifestyle and reduce the risk of relapse;
- enlist and advise on support for continued recovery, including referral to other agencies.

Pharmacological interventions may be used to:

- assist with safe withdrawal/detoxification from alcohol prior to treatment;
- address nutritional deficits;
- prevent relapse.

The time-limited nature of specialist treatment therefore encourages the individual to access supports, including other services, which will assist in maintaining harm-free drinking or abstinence beyond treatment.

The evidence base for treatment interventions

In the UK Orford and Edward's (1977) classic treatment-outcome study had a major impact on views about the nature and effectiveness of treatment. In their study a hundred married male alcoholics were randomly assigned to either a comprehensive three-hour assessment, including goal-setting for abstinence, or to the optimum NHS treatment for alcohol dependence, which involved access to in-patient facilities, psychiatrists and social workers. At follow-up twelve and twenty-four months later, the outcomes for drinking for both groups were identical. This finding confirmed that more treatment did not necessarily result in better outcome. Whilst the amount of treatment offered made no difference, client characteristics (marital cohesion, self-esteem and job status) were predictive of success, or otherwise, at follow-up. Such client characteristics are synonymous with the notion of recovery capital in problem drinkers, whether or not they access treatment. No significant difference was noted in drinking outcome between in-patients and out-patients.

This body of research, in addition to subsequent replications, had a profound effect on the nature of specialist treatment for alcohol problems and prompted a shift from lengthy to brief in-patient services and additionally towards community-based and out-patient services in the UK. From the mid 1970s to the mid 1990s the research literature on treatment effectiveness concluded that structured treatments for alcohol-related problems produced superior results, in most cases, when compared with 'control' groups. In other words treatment was better than nothing. However, the literature also demonstrated that no psychosocial intervention was superior to any other intervention. Four logical responses to these findings emerge:

- the need to review the overall impact of treatment interventions;
- if some treatment interventions are more effective for clients with certain characteristics, then the next step would be to conduct 'client-treatment matching studies';
- the similarity in treatment outcomes points to common processes of change inherent in all psychosocial interventions, irrespective of theoretical basis, mirroring unassisted change;
- consideration of the role of pharmacological interventions in assisting change.

These will be all explored.

Treatment-outcome research reviews

There have been a number of reviews of treatment outcome conducted in the early twenty-first century, based in different countries, all with the overall aim of summarising the evidence for the effectiveness of treatment interventions for moderate to severe alcohol dependence. Three of these reviews are used here, two of which were conducted in the UK.

The Mesa Grande meta-analysis (Miller *et al.*, 2003) consisted of a review of 381 treatment-outcome studies covering a considerable range of specific interventions. Studies were evaluated on the basis of their methodological rigour and ranked accordingly — the 'gold standard' being 'randomised controlled trials' (RCT). In addition, the number of studies on a particular intervention or treatment was taken into account, thus demonstrating the consistency of the intervention over time and across treatment settings. The result is a ranking, which serves to offer guidance in terms of the weight of the evidence. Particular treatments, which may have many adherents, are not featured in the Mesa Grande listing if research of an acceptable standard, or in sufficient volume, has not been carried out: for example, until quite recently there were almost no RCTs conducted on Twelve Step/Alcoholics Anonymous and as a result a relatively low Mesa Grande ranking is allocated. By the same token a significant number of interventions belonging to the 'cognitive behavioural' family of interventions are ranked highly because of the high volume of 'gold standard' studies conducted. The large number of well-conducted studies on cognitive behavioural interventions may serve to skew the overall evidence base and reflect the hegemony of the psychology discipline.

For the Health Technology Board for Scotland (HTBS), Slattery *et al.* (2003) conducted a systematic review of the available scientific treatment literature, 'evidence from experts and professional groups, manufacturers and other interested parties'. The review sought to identify which treatments (psychosocial and pharmacological) would yield the maximum maintenance of recovery amongst those dependent on alcohol, who had been detoxified and were newly abstinent and were therefore ready to engage with relapse-prevention-focused interventions.

The NTA review (Raistrick *et al.*, 2006) takes its lead from Mesa Grande (Miller *et al.*, 2003) and HTBS (Slattery *et al.*, 2003) in providing a perspective on evidence-informed treatments, taking account of both drinking culture and service structures in the UK. Consequently, the review takes a broader approach than either Mesa Grande or HTBS and opts for less restrictive approaches to treatment in the UK. The NTA review (Raistrick *et al.*, 2006) has cast its net wide in its recommendations for evidence-based interventions for alcohol-related problems, which is reflected in NICE (2011) for younger people.

Treatment matching

The most important of these kinds of study are Project MATCH (Babor and Del Boca, 2003) — conducted in the USA and the largest evaluation of psychotherapeutic interventions ever undertaken — and UKATT (2008). As the interventions being tested in both studies had a demonstrated record of effectiveness, control groups were not a feature of the research design. In MATCH three interventions were compared and delivered in a manualised format in order to minimise therapist differences. The goal in all three interventions was abstinence:

- cognitive behavioural therapy (CBT): a coping skills intervention, based on social learning theory, delivered in twelve sessions over twelve weeks;
- Twelve Step Facilitation (TSF): designed to increase access and AA attendance; delivered in twelve sessions over twelve weeks;
- motivational enhancement therapy (MET): based on cognitive and motivational psychology and delivered in four sessions over a twelve-week period.

The findings of Project MATCH surprised the alcohol treatment research field as the 'matching' of client characteristics to intervention hypotheses was not supported. Despite this, some findings have significant implications for the treatment of alcohol dependence:

- CBT was more effective than TSF where individuals had high levels of mental health symptoms. This makes sense given that high levels of psychopathology may make group attendance and interaction extremely difficult for an individual. By the same token an individual whose behaviour is perceived as 'strange' by a group may be less well accepted by its membership.
- TSF was more effective for individuals with social or friendship networks which supported heavy drinking. The importance of AA as the provider of an extensive non-drinking environment and social network is central to moving away from old drinking cues and forging a new way of life, particularly among those who are highly dependent on alcohol.
- MET was more effective than CBT and TSF for individuals who demonstrated high levels of anger. The structure of MET facilitated the expression of current concerns about drinking. MET achieved equivalent outcomes in four sessions compared to twelve for CBT and TSF), consequently delivering a more cost-effective outcome; this was also confirmed by UKATT.
- CBT was more effective than TSF for those who were low in dependence and in turn those highly dependent did better with TSF. Among those with higher levels of dependence the greater

need for non-drinking environments, such as AA, in order to maintain abstinence, is emphasised. More moderate levels of dependence might allow change based on the development of effective planning and coping skills. CBT may then fit well with 'controlled drinking' goals, though the treatment aim in MATCH was abstinence.

Despite the failure to confirm or support the hypothesised 'matches', Project MATCH is very important in developing an understanding of treatment for alcohol dependence. It is the first time in which a Twelve Step intervention has been compared, through random allocation of subjects, to MET and TSF, both of which can be considered mainstream interventions based on psychological theories. As TSF was staffed predominantly by 'recovering alcoholics' the claim that 'only an alcoholic can help an alcoholic' is not supported, given the equivalence of outcomes.

UKATT (2008) is the most important alcohol treatment study in the UK for quite some time, and it sought to explore the implications of Project MATCH for British services (Raistrick *et al.*, 2006). It set out to compare the established effectiveness of an 'extended brief intervention', MET and the social behaviour network therapy (SBNT) designed specifically for the trial. Matching hypotheses were identical in both UKATT and MATCH. MET and SBNT showed equivalent outcomes and the UKATT research team concluded 'that client–treatment matching … is unlikely to result in substantial improvements to the effectiveness of treatment for alcohol problems' (UKATT, 2008, p. 228).

The implications of 'matching' studies are that, despite significant theoretical differences between the interventions studied in MATCH and UKATT, there appear to be few differences in treatment outcome as measured by abstinence or levels of alcohol consumption, resulting in choice of intervention. However, based on matching study findings, levels of dependence, heavy drinking networks, degrees of anger and mental health symptoms may give pointers to appropriate interventions. Both MATCH and UKATT underline the importance of providing well-structured and manualised interventions, delivered by well-trained staff. However, the issue of matching services to client characteristics does not rest there. There are other ways in which treatment seekers are matched to services. In the absence of treatment matching to client characteristics, UKATT (2008) reinforces the importance of clinical/professional judgement in relation to creating treatment interventions that meet the needs of the service user, including the need for on-going support after treatment (SMACAP, 2011). In service delivery settings, whether health or social care oriented, the theme of clinical or professional judgement based on an assessment of individual need is fundamental to matching client need to the interventions and services required. This may be seen as an element of the client–therapist alliance.

Treatment-outcome similarity

Treatment-outcome comparison studies produce similar results. There are a number of factors that may contribute to the similarity in outcome across differing treatments. Some of these influences are a function of the research design and procedures, whilst others are aspects of the treatment setting and the client–therapist 'therapeutic alliance'.

Despite theoretical differences there are potent common ingredients in the treatments interventions tested in MATCH and UKATT, which may explain the similarities in outcome. For example CBT, which focuses on coping skill development, will also support motivation to change and enhance self-belief, both of which are substantial elements of MET. Similarly, TSF, as evidenced by AA attendance, will support motivation, provide direct coping advice ('one day at a time') and provide a non-drinking social environment. Nevertheless, the 'equal outcome' phenomenon has been a feature of general psychotherapy outcome research for a variety of psychotherapeutic interventions (Berglund, 2005).

Problem drinkers who have mental health, homelessness or polydrug use issues are often excluded from treatment-outcome research as these vulnerable characteristics make them more difficult to follow up. The exclusion of the more difficult or troubled individuals makes the remaining subjects more homogenous and limits the generalisability of findings to more vulnerable service users. The selection process for treatment-outcome studies tends to be rigorous and may involve several hours of assessment for study inclusion, prior to administration of the intervention being tested. Assessment for Project MATCH exceeded five hours, whilst by comparison MET in both MATCH and UKATT amounted to no more than four hours. It is feasible that a comprehensive assessment for the purpose of inclusion, or exclusion, from a research project may equate to a treatment intervention in terms of outcome. Furthermore, such assessment will be given to all subjects, irrespective of treatment or control group allocation, and this may limit or obscure measurable differences between the interventions being tested and control conditions. It is proposed by Berglund (2005) and Orford (2008) that the RCT has reached the end of its usefulness in behavioural research on treatment for alcohol problems, and that research should focus on change processes using qualitative methodologies.

The idea of common processes across all treatments also has strong support and a contrary perspective is proposed by Orford who concludes 'that apparently contrasting treatments are, in most respects, not different at all' (Orford, 2008, p. 875). Psychotherapeutic treatment-outcome research concludes that active ingredients are attributed to 'general' factors (Berglund, 2005; Orford, 2008). This is consistent with a change and recovery perspective where a wide range of life factors have primacy, in influencing both change and its maintenance, over the technology of specialist treatment.

Treatment trials by definition attempt to control therapist variables or characteristics by training therapists to a consistent level and also by using treatment manuals as a means of demonstrating the impact of the treatment alone. A key feature of the competent practitioner, in relation to such judgement is their ability to create a therapeutic alliance with the service user. Therapist characteristics (empathy, supportiveness, goal directed and promotion of self-determination) and the therapeutic alliance are important and commonly reported by treatment subjects at follow-up — more so than the particular intervention technique tested (Saunders and Kershaw, 1979; Orford 2008).

The understanding of client need and the ability to be flexible, and effectively deviate from a prescribed treatment intervention, in some respects mirrors the therapeutic alliance associated with positive treatment outcome. Therapist characteristics are an important ingredient in treatment delivery and may account for up to 50% of outcome. 'After all, a half century of psychotherapy research has demonstrated that the most robust predictor of treatment success is the quality of the therapeutic alliance' (Nilsen, 2010, p. 965). These factors contribute to what is perceived as a credible treatment, or service, by the service user, as well as being given attention and a sense of hope. Berglund (2005) further proposes that this experience at the beginning of treatment may explain why single and brief interventions have a potent impact on some subjects over more lengthy interventions.

Pharmacological interventions

The main functions of pharmacological interventions are safe withdrawal from alcohol, the treatment of vitamin deficiency by nutritional supplement and relapse prevention or support for sustained recovery. Medication must be consumed if it is to have any effect; consequently, studies on the effectiveness of medications to treat alcohol-related problems consist of a substantial psychosocial input designed to motivate and support drug compliance. In this section the evidence for the use of pharmacological interventions will be considered including research on combined psychosocial and pharmacological interventions. There are three pharmacological approaches, which are relevant to treatment for alcohol dependence: detoxification, nutritional supplementation and relapse prevention.

Detoxification

Many dependent drinkers stop by themselves without the aid of medication. The process of achieving an alcohol-free state may involve the individual experiencing uncomfortable withdrawal symptoms. Those in contact with medical services and seeking specialist treatment for an alcohol problem may be offered detoxification medication, the emphasis being on safety. Detoxification is achieved rapidly, commonly in 5–10 days, whereby withdrawal symptomatology (e.g. sweats, nausea, tremors) is minimised and serious medical complications (e.g. withdrawal seizures, dementia tremens) are prevented. The drug of choice for detoxification is chlordiazepoxide (Librium), which is a benzodiazepine. However, benzodiazepine prescribing is restricted to the withdrawal period, as further use tends to increase tolerance and dependence in addition to interactions with alcohol

(NICE, 2010b). The achievement of detoxification is commonly a starting point for 'treatment' and is viewed as a requirement for relapse prevention (Slattery *et al.*, 2003). 'The use of benzodiazepines in this manner revolutionised the treatment of alcohol withdrawal and unequivocally reduced the risk of death associated with detoxification' (O'Malley and Kosten, 2006, p. 243).

Nutritional supplements

Thiamine deficiency is a feature of heavy drinking where poor diet is a feature. Wernicke's encephalopathy is a serious consequence of thiamine deficiency (symptoms: confusion, ophthalmoplegia and ataxia) and is treatable by thiamine booster. Failure to spot and treat Wernicke's will result in Korsakoff's syndrome where alcohol-related brain damage (ARBD) is evident in serious and enduring memory loss.

Medications for relapse prevention

Disulfiram

This is a 'sensitising' medication which produces a negative reaction by interfering with liver enzymes in the breakdown of acetaldehyde, when consumed prior to alcohol consumption. Symptoms such as headache, vomiting nausea, flushing and tachycardia are produced.

The noxious symptoms produced by disulfiram in conjunction with alcohol are best thought of in behavioural terms whereby the expected positive outcomes from drinking are altered to being negative, when alcohol is consumed. The individual's knowledge of the reaction and their commitment to taking the medication are crucial and over time the negative expectancies of consuming alcohol following ingestion of disulfiram develop. Where disulfiram is shown to be effective, administration is commonly supervised by a relative or programme staff (O'Malley and Kosten, 2006) and is a central element of the Community Reinforcement Approach (Meyer and Miller, 2001). Disulfiram's purpose then is to maintain abstinence from alcohol and prevent relapse. It also has a similar effect on cocaine use, though by different mechanisms. Disulfiram is recommended by Mesa Grande, HTBS, NTA and NICE.

Acamprosate

This may reduce the physiological and psychological distress and urges (or cravings) to drink which result from alcohol withdrawal and are cued by environmental stimuli. O'Malley and Kosten (2006) report a meta-analysis of seventeen studies involving 4,087 subjects and conclude that abstinence rates at six months were significantly higher in the acamprosate-treated group when compared to a control group given a placebo. However, Slattery *et al.* (2003) note in a European study the limited impact on a Scottish cohort of dependent drinkers, proposing that the pattern of drinking, including binge drinking, may have been a contributory influence. Acamprosate is recommended by Mesa Grande, HTBS, NTA and NICE.

Naltrexone

This is an opioid antagonist, which blocks the effect of opioid drugs such as heroin or methadone at the receptor sites in the central nervous system. It is commonly used to reverse opioid overdose and may block some of the reinforcing or pleasurable effects of alcohol and thereby reduce the risk of relapse to heavy drinking. Naltrexone has been investigated in fifteen studies involving 2,300 alcohol-dependent individuals, with the majority of the studies demonstrating an improved outcome over a placebo treatment (O'Malley and Kosten, 2006). It is recommended by Mesa Grande (Miller *et al.*, 2003) and NICE (2010b).

Combining pharmacological and cognitive behavioural interventions

Whilst evidence exists supporting both the benefits of psychosocial interventions and the use of medication, few studies have investigated the combined effect. In Project COMBINE Anton *et al.* (2006) tested the impact of two relapse-prevention medications — naltrexone and acamprosate — in a variety of combinations with a package of cognitive behavioural interventions including motivational interviewing, coping skills, community support and TSF described as 'combined behavioural intervention'. COMBINE findings demonstrated that both naltrexone and acamprosate showed minor benefits over the placebo and control groups, when combined with CBI (combine behavioural intervention). Naltrexone was most suitable for individuals who have lapsed or slipped, therefore preventing a move towards heavy drinking, while acamprosate appeared to be most suitable for supporting abstinence in those who were concerned that craving would lead to relapse (Anton *et al.*, 2006; Raistrick *et al.*, 2006; NICE, 2010b).

Overall, despite the modest improvements attributable to pharmacological interventions it is likely that the pharmaceutical industry, globally, will continue to develop and evaluate the impact of drugs on ameliorating alcohol problems.

Conclusions

According to Di Clemente (2006, p. 92) treatment is 'a time-limited, circumscribed experience that interacts with and hopefully enhances the self-change process on the road to recovery'. Some people opt for treatment as a result of previous unsuccessful attempts at unassisted change, as part of their recovery process, reflecting the extent of health and social harms which have accrued. Change processes transcend natural recoverers and treatment seekers alike. This confirms important similarities between these overlapping populations and reflects the range of factors, beyond treatment, which influence change and recovery from alcohol problems. Treatment has its place in the recovery journey, for some, and its effectiveness has been demonstrated.

The conclusions from both UK reviews — NTA (Raistrick *et al.*, 2006) and HTBS (Slattery *et al.*, 2003) — are consistent with Mesa Grande findings (Miller *et al.*, 2003) and reflect Miller's (2001) comments on the 'menu of potentially effective treatment methods with which to help clients who have alcohol problems'. This gives a strong pointer to the nature and type of interventions supported and by implication the nature of evidence-based services. Given the similarities in healthcare provision across the UK the HTBS and NTA recommendations are of particular importance. The weight of evidence lies with the cognitive behavioural family of interventions. 'Superiority' for MET is proposed on the basis of equality of drinking outcome with significantly fewer therapist contacts (Raistrick *et al.*, 2006). MET will emerge as a key element in UK treatment services, whereby scarce staff resources can be used to best advantage, reflecting a stepped care perspective to individual need (Scottish Advisory Committee on Drug Misuse, 2008; SMACAP, 2011). However, this may obscure the potential use of less well-researched interventions, particularly given the equity of outcome. Thus the range of effective interventions may be greater than NTA's recommendations.

The findings which underpin evidence-informed practice support structured treatment interventions, with sound theoretical support being delivered by highly trained, competent and committed staff, in well-organised and supportive service settings. Ensuring that therapist skills and therapeutic alliances are maximised is central. Professional and clinical judgement are still required, reflecting the ethos of SMACAP (2011), which advocates a person-centred, recovery-focused approach ensuring that individual needs are identified and met. Importantly mutual self-help is featured, particularly Twelve Step organisations (see Chapter 5) as a recovery vehicle its own right or as post-treatment support for recovery. Medication can make an important contribution in relation to safer detoxification and the resolution of nutritional deficiencies. With regard to relapse prevention there is evidence of modest improvements in outcome when medication is used as adjunct to psychosocial interventions, but not as a replacement. Nor is medication to prevent relapse required in all cases.

No preferred treatment intervention method has been identified and the failure to distinguish between a significant number of interventions has resulted in the view that there is a considerable choice available. In criticising this Orford (2008) calls for treatment research to shift focus from 'techniques' towards investigating processes of change, including common processes across treatments:

> In short, people move in and out of different drinking behaviours and change is best conceptualised as a process, which may or may not be treatment assisted. Certainly there are many social influences that have greater potency than treatment. (Raistrick *et al.*, 2006)

Final summary

It is commonly suggested that the problem with alcohol in Scotland is 'the culture'. There are many ways to change culture. Drinking culture is not static and has evolved during the last half century by bending towards commercial interests resulting in cheaper alcohol and easy access, which is heavily promoted and broadly supported by public and political opinion. Alcohol purchase and consumption have shifted from licensed premises to off-sales purchase and consumption at home, or in public. The health and social problems associated with alcohol require a range of policy responses nationally and locally, including services for individuals. This book has looked at those approaches with the greatest evidence of effectiveness.

It is clear that those living in deprived circumstances suffer more than those who are more affluent, even when they may consume less alcohol. Deprivation appears to underpin many alcohol-related consequences and in turn heavy drinking appears to exacerbate poverty.

Alcohol needs to be more expensive and less available in order to reduce consumption and its health and social consequences. This may come about by a public health policy of increasing and regulating the price of alcohol. Scottish Government has introduced the Alcohol (Minimum Pricing) Bill (2011) and embarked on a consultation process in order to confirm a minimum unit price. Alcohol may become more expensive in relative terms owing to current economic circumstances, which may explain the downturn in consumption in the last few years.

With regard to regulating the drinking environment liquor licensing law has taken on a public health remit. At this stage it is unclear how that will be implemented. Despite this development relaxed licensing hours have been retained, in order to acknowledge wider interests. Therefore, easy access to alcohol will remain though measures to regulate outlets, enforce laws and foster community participation have been enhanced.

At an individual level the means to assist people to change their drinking must be developed. This recognises that many people change, or recover, without formal help, but do require supportive circumstances in order to do so, whether in their family or broader social networks. A significant range of effective interventions are available, which may be deployed in many different settings, including brief interventions. The integration of these approaches across health and social care is less clear, given organisational constraints. Professional reluctance to engage with alcohol problems needs to be tackled by employers and professional bodies alike in order that problem drinkers are not subject to discrimination.

Whilst alcohol production and sale are major elements of the Scottish economy, the impact on society is profound. There is much to be saved, including lives and families, by tackling alcohol problems.

REFERENCES

Acheson, D. (1998) *Independent Inquiry into Inequalities in Health*, London: The Stationery Office. Available at URL: www.dh.gov.uk/en/ Publicationsandstatistics/Publications/PublicationsPolicyAndGuidance/ DH_4097582 (accessed 7 October 2011)

AFS (2009) *Licensing for Public Health*, Glasgow: Alcohol Focus Scotland

Alcohol Commission (2010) *The Report of the Alcohol Commission*, Edinburgh: Scottish Parliament. Available at URL: www.jackiebaillie. co.uk/uploads/13438f00-3097-f2f4-1d07-c4bbbe270c51.pdf (accessed 27 September 2011)

Andreas, J. and O'Farrell, T. (2009) 'Alcoholics anonymous attendance following Twelve Step treatment participation as a link between alcohol-dependent fathers' treatment involvement and their children's externalising problems', *Addiction Research*, Vol. 36, pp. 87–100

Anton, R., O'Malley, S., Ciraulo, D., Cisler, R. *et al.* (2006) 'Combined pharmacotherapies and behavioural interventions for alcohol dependence. The COMBINE study: A randomised controlled trial', *Journal of American Medical Association*, Vol. 293

Babor, T., Caetano, R., Casswell, S., Edwards, G. *et al.* (2003) *Alcohol: No Ordinary Commodity: Research and Public Policy*, Oxford: Oxford University Press

Babor, T. and Del Boca, F. (eds) (2003) *Treatment Matching in Alcoholism*, Cambridge: Cambridge University Press

Babor, T., Higgins-Biddle, J., Dauser, D., Burleson, J. *et al.* (2006) 'Brief interventions for at-risk drinking: Patient outcomes and cost-effectiveness in managed care organisations', *Alcohol and Alcoholism*, Vol. 41, No. 6, pp. 624–31

Barber, J. and Crisp, B. (1995) 'The "pressure to change" approach to with the partners of heavy drinkers', *Addiction*, Vol. 90, pp. 269–76

Barrie, K. (1990) 'Helping in groups', in Collins, S. (ed.) (1990) *Alcohol, Social Work and Helping*, London: Routledge

Barrie, K. (1991) 'Motivational counselling in groups', in Davidson, R., Rollnick, S. and McEwan, I. (eds) (1991) *Counselling Problem Drinkers. New Directions in the Study of Alcohol Group*, London: Routledge

Barrie, K. (1992) 'Professional training', in Plant, M., Ritson, B. and Robertson, R. (eds) (1992) *Alcohol and Drugs: The Scottish Experience*, Edinburgh: Edinburgh University Press

Beale, S., Sanderson, D., Kruger, J., Glanville, J. and Duffy, S. (2009) *The Societal Cost of Alcohol Misuse in Scotland in 2007*, Research Findings, No. 89, Edinburgh: Scottish Government. Available at URL: http://scotland.gov.uk/ Publications/2009/12/29122804/0 (accessed 27 September 2011)

Berglund, M. (2005) 'A better widget? Three lessons for improving addiction treatment from a meta-analytical study', *Addiction*, Vol. 100

Best, D., Rome, A., Hanning, K., White, W. *et al.* (2010) *Research for Recovery: A Review of the Drugs Evidence Base*, Edinburgh: Scottish Government. Available at URL: www.scotland.gov.uk/Publications/2010/08/18112230/0 (accessed 27 September 2011)

Betty Ford Consensus Panel (2007) 'What is recovery? A working definition from the Betty Ford Institute', *Journal of Substance Abuse Treatment*, Vol. 33, pp. 221–8

Bien, T., Miller, W. and Tonigan, S. (1993) 'Brief interventions for alcohol problems; A review', *Addiction*, Vol. 88, No. 3, pp. 315–36

Bischof, G., Rumpf, H., Hapke, U., Meyer, C., John, U. (2000) 'Maintenance factors of recovery from alcohol dependence in treated and untreated individuals', *Alcoholism: Clinical and Experimental Research*, Vol. 24, pp. 1773–7

Bischof, G., Rumpf, H., Hapke, U., Meyer, C., John, U. (2003) 'Types of natural recovery from alcohol dependence: A cluster analysis approach', *Addiction*, Vol. 98, pp. 1737–46

Black, H., Gill, J. and Chick, J. (2011) 'The price of a drink: levels of consumption and price paid per unit of alcohol by Edinburgh's ill drinkers with a comparison to wider alcohol sales in Scotland', *Addiction*, Vol. 106, No. 4, pp. 729–36

Booth, A., Meier, P., Stockwell, T., Sutton, A. *et al.* (2008) 'Part A. Systematic reviews', Sheffield: School of Health and Related Research, University of Sheffield

Braiden, G. (2011) 'Warning over alcohol ban on under 21s: SNP could face backlash from young people', *The Herald*, 1 June

Brennan, A., Purshouse, R., Rafia, R., Taylor, K. and Meier, P. (2008) 'Independent review of alcohol pricing and promotion: Part B Results from the Sheffield Alcohol Policy Model', Sheffield: University of Sheffield

Bromley, C. and Shelton, N. (2010) *The Scottish Health Survey: UK Comparisons*, Edinburgh: Scottish Government. Available from URL: www.scotland. gov.uk/Publications/2010/08/31093025/0 (accessed 27 September 2011)

Bruun, K. (1982) *Alcohol Policies in the UK: Report by the Central Policy Review Staff: May 1979*, Stockholm: University of Stockholm

Bruun, K., Edwards, G., Lumio, M., Makela, K. *et al.* (1975) *Alcohol Control Policies in Public Health Perspective*, Vol. 25, New Brunswick, NJ: Finnish Foundation for Alcohol Studies

Bufe, C. (1998) *Alcoholics Anonymous: Cult or Cure*, Tucson: See Sharp Press

Burns, E., Gray, R., Smith, L. (2010) 'Brief screening questionnaires to identify problem drinking during pregnancy: A systematic review', *Addiction*, Vol. 105, pp. 601–14

Carey, K., Carey, M., Henson, J., Maisto, S. and De Martini, K. (2011) 'Brief alcohol interventions for mandated college students: Comparison of face to face counselling and computer delivered interventions', *Addiction*, Vol. 106, No. 3, pp. 528–37

Casswell, S., Quan You, R., Huckle, T. (2011) 'Alcohol's harm to others: Reduced well-being and health status for those with heavy drinkers in their lives',

Addiction, Vol. 106, No. 6

Chaloupka, F. (2009) 'Alcoholic beverage taxes, prices and drinking', *Addiction*, Vol. 104, pp. 191–2

Chang, G., McNamara, T., Orav, E. *et al.* (2005) 'Brief intervention in prenatal alcohol use: A randomised trial', *Obstetrics and Gynecology*, Vol. 105, pp. 991–8

Chick, J., Lloyd, G. and Crombie, E. (1985) 'Counselling problem drinkers in medical wards: a controlled study', *British Medical Journal*, Vol. 290, pp. 965–7

Clayson, C. (1972) *Report of the Departmental Committee on Scottish Licensing Law*, Edinburgh: HMSO

Cobiac, L., Vos, T., Doran, C. and Wallace, C. (2009) 'Cost–effectiveness of interventions to prevent alcohol-related disease and injury in Australia', *Addiction*, Vol. 104, No. 10, pp. 1646–55

Cochrane, R. and Bal, S. S. (1990) 'Patterns of alcohol consumption by Sikh, Hindu and Muslim men in the West Midlands'. *British Journal of Addiction*, Vol. 85, pp. 759–69

Collins, E., Dickson, N., Eynon, C., Kinver, A. and MacLeod, P. (2008) *Drinking and Driving 2007: Prevalence, Decision Making and Attitudes*, Edinburgh: Scottish Government Social Research. Available at URL: www.scotland.gov.uk/Publications/2008/03/04152525/0 (accessed 28 September 2011)

Copello, A. and Orford, J. (2002) 'Addiction and the family: Is it time for services to take notice of the evidence?', *Addiction*, Vol. 97, pp. 1361–63

Copello, A., Templeton, L., Krishnan, M., Orford, J. and Velleman, R. (2000) 'A treatment package to improve primary care services for the relatives of people with alcohol and drug problems', *Addict Res*, Vol. 8, pp. 471–8

Copello, A., Templeton, L., Orford, J., Velleman, R. *et al.* (2009) 'The relative efficacy of two levels of a primary care intervention for family members affected by the addiction problem of a close relative: a randomised trial', *Addiction*, Vol. 104, pp. 49–58

Cox, M. and Klinger, E. (eds) (2004), *Handbook of Motivational Counselling: Concepts, Approaches, and Assessment*, Chichester: John Wiley

Crawford, M., Patton, R., Touquet, R., Drummond, C. *et al.* (2004) 'Screening and referral for brief intervention of alcohol-misusing patients in an emergency department', *The Lancet*, Vol. 364, pp. 1334–9

Davidson, R. (1992) 'Prochaska and Di Clemente's model of change: A case study', *British Journal of Addiction*, Vol. 87, pp. 821–2

Di Clemente, C. (2006) 'Natural change and the troublesome use of substances: a life course perspective', in Miller, W. and Carroll, K. (eds) (2006) *Rethinking Substance Abuse*, New York: Guildford Press

Di Clemente, C. and Prochaska, J. (1998) 'Toward a comprehensive trans-theoretical model of change: Stages of change in the addictive behaviours', in Miller, W. and Heather, N. (eds) (1998) *Treating Addictive Behaviors, Processes of Change*, 2nd edn, New York: Plenum Press, pp 3–24

DOH (1995) *Sensible Drinking: The Report of an Inter-Departmental Working Group*, London: Department of Health. Available at URL: www.dh.gov.uk/en/Publicationsandstatistics/Publications/PublicationsPolicyAndGuidance/DH_4084701 (accessed 7 October 2011)

DOH (1998) *Independent Inquiry into Inequalities in Health Report*, Norwich: The Stationery Office. Available at URL: www.archive.official-documents. co.uk/document/doh/ih/contents.htm (accessed 18 April 2011)

Donaldson, L. and Rutter, P. (2011) 'Commentary on Black *et al.* (2011): Minimum pricing of alcohol — a solution whose time has come', *Addiction*, Vol. 106, No. 4

D'Onofrio, G. and Degutis, L. C. (2005) *Screening and Brief Intervention in the Emergency Department*, Bethesda, MD: National Institute on Alcohol Abuse and Alcoholism. Available at URL: http://pubs.niaaa.nih.gov/publications/arh28–2/63–72.pdf (accessed February 2011)

Driver Vehicle Licensing Authority (www.dvla.gov.uk)

Drummond, C., Deluca, P., Oyefeso, A., Rome, A. *et al.* (2009) *Scottish Alcohol Needs Assessment*, London: Institute of Psychiatry, King's College

Drummond, C., Oyefeso, A., Phillips, T, Cheeta, S. *et al.* (2005) *Alcohol Needs Assessment Research Project (ANARP)*, The 2004 ANARP for England, London: Department of Health

Duffy, J. (1992) 'Scottish licensing reforms', in Plant, M., Ritson, B. and Robertson, R. (eds) (1992) *Alcohol and Drugs: The Scottish Experience*, Edinburgh: Edinburgh University Press

Duffy, T., Holttum, S. and Keegan, M. (1998) 'An investigation of the impact of training social workers and their managers', *Alcoholism*, Vol. 34, Nos 1–2, pp. 93–104

Dunbar, J. (1992) 'Drink and driving', in Plant, M., Ritson, B. and Robertson, R. (eds) (1992) *Alcohol and Drugs: The Scottish Experience*, Edinburgh: Edinburgh University Press

Dunn, C., Deroo, L. and Rivara, F. (2001) 'The use of brief interventions adapted from motivational interviewing across behavioural domains: a systematic review', *Addiction*, Vol. 96, No. 12, pp. 1725–42

Eadie, D., MacAskill, S., Brooks, O. *et al.* (2010) *Pre-teens Learning about Alcohol: Drinking and Family Contexts*, York: Joseph Rowntree Foundation

Edwards, G. (1982) *The Treatment of Drinking Problems*, London: Blackwell

Edwards, G. (2000) 'Editorial note: Natural recovery is the only recovery', *Addiction*, Vol. 95, No. 5, p. 747

Forrester, D. (2000) 'Parental substance misuse and child protection in a British sample', *Child Abuse Review*, Vol. 9, No. 4

Galvani, S. and Forrester, D. (2011) *Social Work Services and Recovery from Substance Misuse: A Review of the Evidence*, Edinburgh: Scottish Government Social Research. Available at URL: http://scotland.gov.uk/Publications/2011/03/18085806/0 (accessed 28 September 2011)

Gartner, A. (2009) *Alcohol and Health: A Profile of Alcohol and Health in Wales*, Cardiff: Wales Centre for Health. Available at URL: www.wales. nhs.uk/sites3/Documents/568/Alcohol%20and%20Health%20in%20 Wales_WebFinal_E.pdf (accessed 28 September 2011)

GCPH (2007) *Comparisons of Health-Related Behaviours and Health Measures between Glasgow and the Rest of Scotland*, Briefing Paper 7, Glasgow: Glasgow Centre for Population Health

GCPH (2010) Investigating a 'Glasgow Effect': Why Do Equally Deprived UK

Cities Experience Different Health Outcomes?, Briefing Paper 25, Glasgow: Glasgow Centre for Population Health

Geisbrecht, N., Cukier, S. and Steeves, D. (2010) 'Collateral damage from alcohol: implications of "second-hand effects of drinking" for populations and health priorities', *Addiction*, Vol. 105, pp. 1323–5

Gentilello, L., Rivara, F., Donovan, D., Jurkovich, G. *et al.* (1999) 'Alcohol interventions in a trauma center as a means of reducing the risk of injury recurrence', *Annals of Surgery*, Vol. 230, No. 4, p. 473

Gilchrist, G., Moskalewicz, J., Slezakova, S., Okruhlica, L. *et al.* (2011) 'Staff regard towards working with substance users: a European multi-centre study', *Addiction*, Vol. 106, No. 6, pp. 1114–25

Gmel, G., Kuntsche, E. and Rehm, J. (2011) 'Risky single-occasion drinking: Bingeing is not bingeing', *Addiction*, Vol. 106, No. 6

Gossop, M., Stewart, D. and Marsden, J. (2008) 'Attendance at Narcotics Anonymous and Alcoholics Anonymous meetings, frequency of attendance and substance-use outcomes after residential treatment for drug dependence: A five year follow-up study', *Addiction*, Vol. 103, No. 1

Granfield, R. and Cloud, W. (1999) *Coming Clean: Overcoming Addiction Without Treatment*, New York: New York University Press

Gray, L. (2007) *Comparisons of Health-Related Behaviours and Health Measures Between Glasgow and the Rest of Scotland*, Glasgow: Glasgow Centre for Population Health. Available at URL: www.gcph.co.uk/publications/108_findings_series_7-health-related_behaviours_and_measures (accessed 7 October 2011)

Griesbach, D., Lardner, C. and Russell, P. (2009) *Managing the Needs of Drunk and Incapable People in Scotland: A literature Review and Needs Assessment*, Edinburgh: Scottish Government Social Research. Available at URL: www.scotland.gov.uk/Publications/2009/10/29154403/4 (accessed 28 September 2011)

Hanlon, P., Walsh, D. and Whyte, B. (2006) *Let Glasgow Flourish*, Glasgow: Glasgow Centre for Population Health

Harbin, F. and Murphy, M. (eds) (2000) *Substance Misuse and Child Care: How to Understand, Assist and Intervene When Drugs Affect Parenting*, Lyme Regis: Russell House Publishing

Harkins, C. and Poley, D. (2011) 'Making Alcohol Policy: Increasing consumption or reducing harm', *Alcohol Alert*, Vol. 1, pp. 20–2

Harris, J., Best, D., Gossop, M., Marshall, J. *et al.* (2003) 'Prior Alcoholics Anonymous (AA) affiliation and the acceptability of the Twelve Steps to patients entering UK statutory addiction treatment', *Journal of Studies on Alcohol*, Vol. 64

Hodgson, R., John, B., Abbasi, T., Hodgson, R. C. *et al.* (2003) 'Fast screening for alcohol misuse', *Addictive Behaviours*, Vol. 28, pp. 1453–63

Holder, H. (2007) 'What we learn from a reduction in the retail alcohol prices: Lessons from Finland', *Addiction*, Vol. 102

Home Office (2003) *Guidance for Local Partnerships on Alcohol-Related Crime and Disorder Data*, Development and Practice Report 6. London: Home Office. Available at URL: http://webarchive.nationalarchives.gov.

uk/20110218135832/http://rds.homeoffice.gov.uk/rds/pdfs2/dpr6.pdf (accessed 28 September 2011)

Home Office (2010) *2010 Drug Strategy Consultation Paper*. London: Home Office. Available at URL: www.homeoffice.gov.uk/publications/consulta-tions/cons-drug-strategy-2010/drugs-consultation?view=Binary (accessed 4 October 2011)

Homel, R., McIlwain, G. and Carvolth, R. (2004) 'Creating safer drinking environments', in Heather, N. and Stockwell, T. (eds) (2004) *The Essential Handbook of Treatment and Prevention of Alcohol Problems*, Chichester: Wiley

House of Commons Health Committee (2010) *First Report: Alcohol*, London: The Stationery Office. Available at URL: www.publications.parliament.uk/pa/cm200910/cmselect/cmhealth/151/15102.htm (accessed 4 October 2011)

Humphreys, K. (2006) 'The trials of Alcoholics Anonymous', *Addiction*, Vol. 101, pp. 617–18

Humphreys, K. and Moos, R. (1996) 'Reduced substance abuse related health-care costs among voluntary participants of AA', *American Psychiatric Association*, Vol. 47

Humphreys, K., Moos, R. and Finney, J. (1995) 'Two pathways out of drink-ing problems without professional treatment', *Addictive Behaviours*, Vol. 20, No. 4

Humphreys, K. and Noke, J. (1997) 'The influence of post-treatment mutual help group participation on the friendship networks of substance abuse patients', *American Journal of Community Psychology*, Vol. 25, No. 1

ISD (2009) *Alcohol Statistics Scotland 2009*, Edinburgh: NHS National Services Scotland. Available at URL: www.alcoholinformation.isdscot-land.org/alcohol_misuse/files/alcohol_stats_bul_09.pdf (accessed 28 September 2011)

ISD (2011) *Alcohol Statistics Scotland 2011*, Edinburgh: NHS National Ser-vices Scotland. Available at URL: www.alcoholinformation.isdscotland.org/alcohol_misuse/files/alcohol_stats_bulletin_2011_updated_110413.pdf (accessed 28 September 2011)

Jenkins, R., Lewis, P., Bebbington, T. *et al.* (1997) 'The national psychiatric morbidity surveys of Great Britain — Initial findings from the household survey', *Psychological Medicine*, Vol. 27, pp. 775–89

Kaner, E., Heather, N., McAvoy, B., Lock, C. and Gilvarry, E. (1999) 'Interven-tion for excessive alcohol consumption in primary healthcare: Attitudes and practices of English general practitioners', *Alcohol and Alcoholism*, Vol. 34, pp. 559–66

Kaner, E., Locke, C., Heather, N., McNamee, P. and Bond, S. (2002) 'Promoting brief alcohol intervention by nurses in primary care: a cluster randomised controlled trial', *Patient Education and Counselling*, Vol. 51, No. 3, pp. 277–84

Kaskutas, L., Bond, J. and Humphreys, K. (2002) 'Social networks as mediators of the effect of AA', *Addiction*, Vol. 97, No. 7

Kendell, R., De Roumanie, M. and Ritson, B. (1983) 'Influence of an increase in excise duty on alcohol consumption and its adverse effects', *British Medical Journal*, Vol. 287, pp. 809–11

Klingemann, H. (2004) 'Natural recovery from alcohol problems', in Heather,

N. and Stockwell, T. (eds) (2004) *The Essential Handbook of Treatment and Prevention of Alcohol Problems*, Chichester: Wiley

Koski, A., Siren, R., Vuori, E. and Poikolainen, K. (2007) 'Alcohol tax cuts and increase in alcohol–positive sudden deaths — a time-series intervention analysis', *Addiction*, Vol. 102

Kypri, K., Jones, C., McElduff, P. and Barker, D. (2010) 'Effects of restricting pub closing times on night-time assaults in an Australian city', *Addiction*, Vol. 106, pp. 303–10

Laslett, A.-M., Room, R., Ferris, J., Wilkinson, C. *et al.* (2011) 'Surveying the range and magnitude of alcohol's harm to others in Australia', *Addiction*, Vol. 106, No. 9, pp. 1603–11

Laudet, A. B. and White, W. L. (2008) 'Recovery capital as prospective predictor of sustained recovery, life-satisfaction and stress among former poly-substance users', *Substance Use and Misuse*, Vol. 43, No. 1, pp. 27–54

Leonard, K. (2011) 'Commentary on Livingston (2011): Alcohol outlets and domestic violence — acute effects and the social ecology of neighbourhoods may both contribute to the relationship', *Addiction*, Vol. 106, No. 5, pp. 926–7

Lightfoot, P. and Orford, J. (1986) 'Helping agents' attitudes towards alcohol-related problems: Situations vacant? A test and elaboration of a model', *British Journal of Addiction*, Vol. 81, No. 6, pp. 749–56

Livingston, M. (2011) 'A longitudinal analysis of alcohol outlet density and domestic violence', *Addiction*, Vol. 106, No. 5, pp. 919–25

Lopez-Quintero, C., Hasin, D., Perez de Los Cobos, J., Pines, A. *et al.* (2011) 'Probability and predictors of remission from lifetime nicotine, alcohol, cannabis and cocaine dependence: Results from the national epidemiologic survey on alcohol and related conditions', *Addiction*, Vol. 106, No. 3, pp. 657–69

Makela, P. and Osterberg, E. (2009) 'Weakening of one more alcohol control pillar: A review of the effects of the alcohol tax cuts in Finland in 2004', *Addiction*, Vol. 104, pp. 554–63

Marks, D., O'Connor, R., Carney, T. and Clarke, A. (2011) 'Added value of applied health psychology: The social and psychological factors contributing to binge drinking in college students', Conference paper, Northampton: University of Northampton

Mayfield, D., McLeod, G. and Hall, P. (1974). 'The CAGE questionnaire: Validation of a new alcoholism screening instrument', *American Journal of Psychiatry*, Vol. 131, pp. 1121–3. Available at URL: http://counsellingresource.com/lib/quizzes/drug-testing/alcohol-cage (accessed 28 September 2011)

McCambridge, J. and Strang, J. (2004) 'The efficacy of a single-session motivational interviewing in reducing drug consumption and perceptions of drug-related risk among young people: Results from a multi-site cluster', *Addiction*, Vol. 99, pp. 39–52

McCambridge, J. and Strang, J. (2005) 'Deterioration over time in effect of motivational interviewing in reducing drug consumption and related risk among young people', *Addiction*, Vol. 100, pp. 470–8

McCartney, G., Collins, C., Walsh, D. and Batty, D. (2011) *Accounting for*

Scotland's Excess Mortality: Towards a Synthesis, Glasgow: Glasgow Centre for Population Health

McPhee, I. (2011) 'How prohibition influences the hidden social worlds of non-treatment-seeking illegal drug users in Scotland', unpublished PhD thesis, Stirling: University of Stirling

Meier, P., Purshouse, R. and Brennan, A. (2010) 'Policy options for alcohol price regulation: The importance of modelling population heterogeneity', *Addiction*, Vol. 105

Mello, M., Nirenberg, T., Longabaugh, R., Woolard *et al.* (2005) 'Emergency department brief motivational interventions for alcohol with motor vehicle crash patients', *Annals of Emergency Medicine*, Vol. 45, No. 6, pp. 620–5

Meyers, R. J. and Miller, W. R. (2001) *A Community Reinforcement Approach to the Treatment of Addiction*, Cambridge: Cambridge University Press

Miller, W. and Carroll, K. (eds) (2006) *Rethinking Substance Abuse: What the Science Shows, and What We Should Do About It*, New York: Guildford Press

Miller, W., Wilbourne, P. and Hettema, J. (2003) 'What works? A summery of alcohol treatment outcome research', in Hester, R. and Miller, W. (eds) (2003) *Handbook of Alcoholism Treatment Approaches: Effective Alternatives*, Boston, MA: Allyn and Bacon

Moore, A., Blow, F., Hoffing, M., Welgreen, S. *et al.* (2011) 'Primary care based intervention to reduce at-risk drinking in older adults: A randomised controlled trial', *Addiction*, Vol. 106, pp. 111–20

Moos, R. (2008) 'Active ingredients of substance-use-focused self-help groups', *Addiction*, Vol. 103, No. 3

Moyer, A., Finney, J., Swearingen, C. and Vergun, P. (2002) 'Brief interventions for alcohol problems: A meta-analytic review of controlled investigations in treatment seeking and non-treatment-seeking populations', *Addiction*, Vol. 97, No. 3, pp. 279–92

Muller, S., Piontek, D., Pabst, A., Baumeister, A. and Kraus, L. (2010) 'Changes in alcohol consumption after the introduction of the alcopops tax in Germany', *Addiction*, Vol. 105

NHS Information Centre (2010) *Statistics on Alcohol: England 2010*, Leeds: Health and Social Care Information Centre. Available at URL: www.ic.nhs.uk/webfiles/publications/alcohol10/Statistics_on_Alcohol_England_2010.pdf (accessed 28 September 2011)

NHS Quality Improvement Scotland (2005), *Clinical Indicators 2005*, Edinburgh: NHSScotland. Available at URL: www.healthcareimprovementscotland.org/previous_resources/indicators/clinical_indicators_2005.aspx (accessed 28 September 2011)

NHSScotland (2006) *Rights Relationships and Recovery*, Edinburgh: Scottish Executive. Available at URL: www.scotland.gov.uk/Publications/2006/04/18164814/0 (accessed 28 September 2011)

NHSScotland (2008) *Alcohol Brief Interventions Training Manual*, Edinburgh: NHSScotland. Available at URL: www.alcoholinformation.isdscotland.org/alcohol_misuse/3932.html (accessed 28 September 2011)

NICE (2010a) *Alcohol-Use Disorders: Preventing the Development of Hazardous and Harmful Drinking*, NICE Public Health Guidance 24, London: NHS

National Institute for Clinical Excellence. Available at URL: www.nice.org.uk/PH24 (accessed 28 September 2011)

NICE (2010b) *Alcohol-use Disorders: Diagnosis and Clinical Management of Alcohol-Related Physical Complications*, NICE Clinical Guidance 100, London: NHS National Institute for Clinical Excellence. Available at URL: www.nice.org.uk/nicemedia/live/12995/48989/48989.pdf (accessed 28 September 2011)

NICE (2011) *Alcohol-use Disorders: Diagnosis, Assessment and Management of Harmful Drinking and Alcohol Dependence*, NICE Clinical Guidance 115. NHS National Institute for Clinical Excellence. Available at URL: www.nice.org.uk/nicemedia/live/13337/53191/53191.pdf (accessed 28 September 2011)

Nicholson Report (2003) *Review of Liquor Licensing Law in Scotland*, Edinburgh: Scottish Executive. Available at URL: www.scotland.gov.uk/Publications/2003/08/17590/22947 (accessed 28 September 2011)

Nilsen, P. (2010) 'Brief alcohol intervention — where to from here? Challenges remain for research and practice', *Addiction*, Vol. 105, pp. 954–9

O'Malley, S. and Kosten, T. (2006) 'Pharmacotherapy of addictive disorders', in Miller, W. and Carroll, K. (eds) (2006) *Rethinking Substance Abuse: What the Science Shows, and What We Should Do About It*, New York: Guildford Press

OPCS (1985) *Drinking and Attitudes to Licensing in Scotland*, OPCS Monitor 55, n.p.: Office of Population Censuses and Surveys

O'Rawe, S. (2006) 'Investigating levels of problem drinking among those on methadone maintenance programmes: implications for individuals and services', MSc Thesis, Paisley: University of the West of Scotland

Orford, J. (2001) *Excessive Appetites: A Psychological View of Addictions*, 2nd edn, Chichester: Wiley

Orford, J. (2008) 'Asking the right questions in the right way: The need for a shift in research on psychological treatments for addiction', *Addiction*, Vol. 103, No. 6, pp. 875–85

Orford, J. and Edwards, G. (1977) *Alcoholism*, Maudsley Monograph 26, Oxford: Oxford University Press

Orford, J., Natera, G., Copello, A., Atkinson, C., *et al.* (2005) *Coping with Alcohol and Drug Problems: The Experiences of Family Members in Three Contrasting Cultures*, London: Routledge

Ouimette, P., Moos, R. and Finney, J. (1998) 'Influence of out-patient treatment and Twelve Step group involvement on on-year substance abuse treatment outcomes', *Journal of Studies on Alcohol*, Vol. 59

Paljarva, T., Koskenvuo, M., Poikolainen, K. *et al.* (2009) 'Binge drinking and depressive symptoms: A 5 year population based cohort study', *Addiction*, Vol. 104, No. 7

Percy, A., Wilson, J., McCartan, C. and McCrystal, P. (2011) *Teenage Drinking Cultures*, York: Joseph Rowntree Foundation. Available at URL: www.jrf.org.uk/sites/files/jrf/teenage-drinking-culture-summary.pdf (accessed 28 September 2011)

Poikolainen, K. (1999) 'Effectiveness of brief interventions to reduce alcohol intake in primary healthcare populations: A meta–analysis', *Preventive Medicine*, Vol. 28, No. 5, pp. 503–9

Professional Social Work (2011) 'Social workers want more drugs and alcohol training', *Professional Social Work*, January. Birmingham: British Association of Social Workers

Raistrick, D., Heather, N. and Godfrey, C. (2006) *Review of the Effectiveness of Treatment for Alcohol Problems*, London: NHS National Treatment Agency for Substance Misuse. Available at URL: www.nta.nhs.uk/uploads/nta_review_of_the_effectiveness_of_treatment_for_alcohol_problems_full-report_2006_alcohol2.pdf (accessed 28 September 2011)

Raistrick, D., Hodgson, R. and Ritson, B. (eds) (1999) *Tackling Alcohol Together: The Evidence Base for a UK Alcohol Policy*, London: Free Association Books

Ray, G., Mertens, J. and Weisner, C. (2009) 'Family members of people with alcohol or drug dependence: Health and medical cost compared to family members of people with diabetes and asthma', *Addiction*, Vol. 104, No. 2

Rehm, J., Bauliunas, D., Borges, G., Graham, K. *et al.* (2010) 'The relation between different dimensions of alcohol consumption and burden of disease: An overview', *Addiction*, Vol. 105

Robertson, I. and Heather, N. (1998) *So You Want to Cut Down Your Drinking? A Self-help Guide to Sensible Drinking*, Edinburgh: Health Education Board Scotland

Robinson, S., Harris, H. and Dunstan, S. (2011) *Smoking and Drinking Among Adults, 2009: A Report on the 2009 General Lifestyle Survey*, Newport: Office for National Statistics

Room, R., Babor, T. and Rehm, J. (2005) 'Alcohol and public health', *Lancet*, Vol. 365, pp. 519–30

Room, R. and Livingston, M. (2010) 'Who drinks how much less with which price policy? A rich feast for policy discussion', *Addiction*, Vol. 105

Room, R. and Rehm, J. (2011) 'Alcohol and non-communicable diseases — cancer heart disease and more', *Addiction*, Vol. 106

Room, R., Rehm, J. and Parry, C. (2011) 'Alcohol and non-communicable diseases (NCDs): Time for a serious international public health effort', *Addiction*, Vol. 106, No. 9

Rumpf, H., Bischof, G., Hapke, U., Meyer, C. and John, U. (2000) 'Studies on natural recovery from alcohol dependence: Sample selection bias by media solicitation?', *Addiction*, Vol. 95, pp. 765–75

Russell, M. (1994) 'New assessment tools for risk drinking during pregnancy: T-ACE, TWEAK and others', *Alcohol Health and Research World*, Vol. 18, pp. 55–61

SALSUS (2008) *Scottish Schools Adolescent Lifestyle and Substance Use Survey (SALSUS). National Report: Smoking, Drinking and Drug Use Among 13 and 15 Year Olds in Scotland in 2008*, Edinburgh: NHSScotland. Available at URL: www.drugmisuse.isdscotland.org/publications/local/SALSUS_2008.pdf (accessed 28 September 2011)

Saunders, W. and Kershaw, P. (1979) 'Spontaneous remission from alcoholism — A community study', *British Journal of Addiction*, Vol. 74, No. 3, pp. 251–65

Schutze, M., Boeing, H., Pischon, T., Rehm, J. *et al.* (2011) 'Alcohol attributable burden of incidence of cancer in eight European countries based on results from prospective cohort study', *British Medical Journal*. Available at URL:

www.bmj.com/content/342/bmj.d1584 (accessed 28 September 2011)

Scottish Advisory Committee on Drug Misuse (2008) *Essential Care: A Report on the Approach Required to Maximise Opportunity for Recovery from Problem Substance Use in Scotland*, Edinburgh: Scottish Government. Available at URL: www.scotland.gov.uk/Publications/2008/03/20144059/0 (accessed 28 September 2011)

Scottish Executive (2002) *Plan for Action on Alcohol Abuse*, Edinburgh, Scottish Executive

Scottish Executive (2003a) *Getting Our Priorities Right: Good Practice Guidance for Working with Children and Families Affected by Substance Misuse*, Edinburgh: Scottish Executive. Available at URL: www.scotland.gov.uk/Publications/2003/02/16469/18705 (accessed 28 September 2011)

Scottish Executive (2003b) *Mind the Gaps: Meeting the Needs of People with Co-Occurring Substance Misuse and Mental Health Problems*, Report of Joint Working Group: SACDM and SACAM, Edinburgh: Scottish Executive. Available from URL: www.scotland.gov.uk/Publications/2003/10/18358/28079 (accessed 28 September 2011)

Scottish Executive (2004) *Off-Sales in the Community. Report of the Working Group on Off-Sales in the Community*, Edinburgh: Scottish Executive. Available from URL: www.scotland.gov.uk/Publications/2004/02/18764/31731 (accessed 28 September 2011)

Scottish Executive (2006) *Getting It Right for Every Child: Implementation Plan*, Edinburgh: Scottish Executive. Available at URL: www.scotland.gov.uk/Publications/2006/06/22092413/0 (accessed 28 September 2011)

Scottish Executive (2007) *Licensing (Scotland) Act 2005. Guidance for Licensing Boards and Local Authorities*, Edinburgh: Scottish Executive. Available from URL: http://scotland.gov.uk/Publications/2007/04/13093458/0 (accessed 28 September 2011)

Scottish Government (2007) *Plan for Action on Alcohol Problems*, Edinburgh: Scottish Government. Available at URL: www.scotland.gov.uk/Publications/2007/02/19150222/0 (accessed 28 September 2011)

Scottish Government (2008a) *The Road to Recovery. A New Approach to Tackling Scotland's Drug Problem*, Edinburgh: Scottish Government. Available at URL: www.scotland.gov.uk/Publications/2008/05/22161610/0 (accessed 28 September 2011)

Scottish Government (2008b) *Equally Well. Report of the Ministerial Task Force on Health Inequalities*, Edinburgh: Scottish Government. Available at URL: www.scotland.gov.uk/Publications/2008/06/09160103/0 (accessed 28 September 2011)

Scottish Government (2008c) *Changing Scotland's Relationship with Alcohol: A Discussion Paper on Our Strategic Approach*, Edinburgh: Scottish Government. Available from URL: www.scotland.gov.uk/Publications/2008/06/16084348/0 (accessed 28 September 2011)

Scottish Government (2009) *A Review of Fixed Penalty Notices (FPN) for Antisocial Behaviour*, Edinburgh: Scottish Government. Available at URL: www.scotland.gov.uk/Publications/2009/11/24155814/4 (accessed 12 August 2011)

Scottish Government (2010a) *National Guidance for Child Protection in Scotland 2010*, Edinburgh: Scottish Government. Available at URL: www.scotland.gov. uk/Publications/2010/12/09134441/0 (accessed 28 September 2011)

Scottish Government (2010b) *The Healthcare Quality Strategy for NHSScotland*, Edinburgh: Scottish Government. Available at URL: www.scotland.gov.uk/ Publications/2010/05/10102307/0 (accessed 28 September 2011)

Scottish Government (2011a) *Drugs and Alcohol — Liquor Licensing: High Level Summary of Statistics Trend Last Update: Monday, 28 March 2011*. Available at URL: www.scotland.gov.uk/Topics/Statistics/Browse/Crime-Justice/Trend-Data (accessed 13 April 2011)

Scottish Government (2011b) Alcohol (Minimum Pricing) (Scotland) Bill. Scottish Government, Edinburgh. Available at URL: http://www.scottish.parliament.uk/S4_Bills/Alcohol%20(Minimum%20Pricing)%20 (Scotland)%20Bill/Bill_as_introduced.pdf

Scottish Government and Convention of Scottish Local Authorities (2010) *Supporting the Development of Scotland's Alcohol and Drug Workforce*, Joint Statement 22 December 2010. Available at URL: www.healthscotland.com/ alcoholanddrug-workforce.aspx (accessed 10 September 2011)

Shaw, S., Cartwright, J. and Harwin, J. (1978) *Responding to Drinking Problems*, London: Croom Helm

SIGN (2003) *Management of Harmful Drinking and Alcohol Dependence in Primary Care*, Guideline 74, Edinburgh: Scottish Inter-Collegiate Guidelines Network. Available at URL: www.sign.ac.uk/pdf/sign74.pdf (accessed 28 September 2011)

Slattery, J., Chick, J., Cochrane, M., Craig, J. *et al.* (2003) *Prevention of Relapse in Alcohol Dependence. Health Technology Assessment Report 3*. Glasgow: Health Technology Board for Scotland

SMACAP (2011) *Quality Alcohol Treatment*, Edinburgh: Scottish Government. Available at URL: www.scotland.gov.uk/Publications/2011/03/21111515/0 (accessed 28 September 2011)

Smith, S., Touquet, R., Wright, S. and Das Gupta, N. (1996) 'Detection of alcohol-misusing patients in accident and emergency departments: The Paddington alcohol test (PAT)', *Journal of Accident and Emergency Medicine*, Vol. 13, pp. 308–12

Sobell, L., Ellingstad, T. and Sobell, M. (2000) 'Natural recovery from alcohol and drug problems: methodological review of the research with suggestions for future directions', *Addiction*, Vol. 95, pp. 749–64

Sokol, R., Martier, S. and Ager, J. (1989) 'The T-ACE questions: Practical prenatal detection of risk-drinking', *American Journal of Obstetrics and Gynecology*, Vol. 160, pp. 863–70

Sondhi, A. and Turner, C. (2011) *The Influence of Family and Friends on Young Peoples Drinking*, York: Joseph Rowntree Foundation

Stockwell, T. and Gruenewald, P. (2004) 'Controls on the Physical Availability of Alcohol', in Heather, N. and Stockwell, T. (eds) (2004) *The Essential Handbook of Treatment and Prevention of Alcohol Problems*, Chichester: Wiley

Stockwell, T., Zhao, J., Macdonald, S., Pakula, B. *et al.* (2009) 'Changes in per capita alcohol sales during the partial privatisation of British Columbia's retail alcohol monopoly 2003–2008: A multi-level local area analysis', *Addiction*, Vol. 104, pp. 1827–36

Thom, B. (1999) *Dealing with Drink. Alcohol and Social Policy: From Treatment to Management*, London: Free Association Books

UKATT (2008) 'UK alcohol treatment trial: Client-treatment matching effects', *Addiction*, Vol. 103

Vaillant, G. E. (1983) *The Natural History of Alcoholism*, Cambridge, MA: Harvard University Press

Vaillant, G. E. (2003) 'A 60-year follow-up of alcoholic men', *Addiction*, Vol. 98, pp. 1043–51

Valentine, G., Jayne, M., Gould, M. and Keenan, J. (2010) *Family Life and Alcohol Consumption: A Study of the Transmission of Drinking Practices*, York: Joseph Rowntree Foundation

Wagenaar, A. (1993). 'Minimum drinking age and alcohol availability to youth: Issues and research needs', in Hilton, M. and Bloss, G. (eds) (1993) *Economics and the Prevention of Alcohol-Related Problems*, Bethesda, MD: National Institute on Alcohol Abuse and Alcoholism

Wagenaar, A. (2010) 'Commentary on Muller *et al.*: Tax policy on alcopops – advances and limitations', *Addiction*, Vol. 105, pp. 1214–15

Wagenaar, A., Salois, M. and Komro, K. (2009) 'Effects of beverage alcohol price and tax levels on drinking: A meta-analysis of 1,003 estimates from 112 studies', *Addiction*, Vol. 104, pp. 179–90

Watson, H., Munro, A., Wilson, M., Kerr, S. and Godwin, J. (2011) *The Involvement of Nurses and Midwives in Screening and Brief Interventions for Hazardous and Harmful Use of Alcohol and Other Psychoactive Substances*, Geneva: World Health Organization

Weaver, T., Madden, P., Charles, V., Stimson, G. *et al.* (2003) 'Co-morbidity of substance misuse and mental illness in community mental health and substance misuse services', *British Journal of Psychiatry*, Vol. 183, pp. 304–13

White, W. (2008) 'The mobilisation of community resources to support long-term addiction recovery', *Journal of Substance Abuse Treatment*, Vol. 362, pp. 146–58

White, W. and Kurtz, E. (2006) *Linking Addiction Treatment and Communities of Recovery: A Primer for Addiction Counselors and Recovery Coaches*, Kansas City, MO: Northeast ATTC

WHO (1992) *The ICD-10 Classification of Mental and Behavioural Disorders*, Geneva: World Health Organization

WHO (1993) *International Statistical Classification of Disease and Health-Related Problems*, ICD 10, Geneva: World Health Organization

WHO (1994) *Lexicon of Alcohol and Drug Terms*, Geneva: World Health Organization

WHO (1996) *Alcohol Use Disorders Identification Test (AUDIT)*, Geneva: World Health Organization. Available at URL: http://whqlibdoc.who.int/hq/2001/who msd msb 01.6a.pdf (accessed 28 September 2011)

WHO (2010) *European Status Report on Alcohol and Health*, Geneva: World Health Organization

Williams, D. (2011) 'Lowdown on the high street', *Observer Food Monthly* No. 119 (April), London: *Observer*

Wilson, G. (1940) *Alcohol and the Nation: A Contribution to the Study of the Liquor Problem in the United Kingdom from 1800 to 1935*, London: Nicholson and Watson

INDEX

Note: page numbers in *italic* denote figures or tables